MADHOUSE

By Robert Goulet

A Howard Greenfeld Book
J. Philip O'Hara, Inc.
Chicago

J. Philip O'Hara, Inc. 20 East Huron, Chicago, 60611. Published simultaneously in Canada by Van Nostrand Reinhold Ltd., Scarborough, Ontario.

LC Number: 72-13318

ISBN: 0-87955- 304-9

First Printing February, 1973

This Book is for Valerie

CHAPTER ONE

It was like one of those nights over Timberland when you cannot trace a single pine in the forestside because there is no strength left to look up after so many strokes of the axe. All was silent, still. Darkness seemed friendly. I tried to sleep.

But sleep soon grew into a sensation of being awake against my will. My head was a throbbing cage of misery, steady blows of pain knocked at my temples, rushes of blood set the skin to burning on my legs. I wondered if someone had hit me on the head. My eyelids felt so heavy I could not open my eyes, see where I was, find a clue to what had happened. Or perhaps I did not want to face yet what now began to dawn on me in nagging darts of recall. I could hear a motor in the night, a steady sound, gentle and near as a friend who promises to do all the straining for you from now on. "Relax," I thought. They were taking me somewhere at last. That was enough to sleep on a while longer.

The engine now roared into a shift in gear. I felt a sudden pull to the left and realized we were rounding a sharp curve to the right. From the rolling of my head I knew I was lying down. But I could not lift my hands, move my feet. An impossible weight held me still. In sudden fear of choking I opened my eyes.

A black holster hung from a stretcher overhead. In the dim light of the vehicle I made out a pair of boots dangling close to the pistol. My head rolled again, as we went into another hairpin curve, then on coming out of it I saw Jesus at the foot of my stretcher. He was trimming his nails and watching me out of the corner of his eye. His black winged cap was on the floor, next to another pair of boots. Sitting at the head of my stretcher was Pepe.

"Quite an escort!" I thought, wondering if it was the Cabo himself lying up there. "Three guardias!" It gave me a pleasant sense of importance. But in a moment I was struck with panic at the thought of why I was here.

My tongue stuck to my palate when I tried to ask them what I had done. I made another effort to free my hands, move my feet, but the straps were too tight. "Jesus," I said.

He stared at me, but seemed not to know who I was. His lips shaped silent words towards Pepe.

Again I made a desperate attempt to say something. But my mouth was a pit of hot, pasty dryness, and all I could hear was a faint noise in my throat, as if chewing for a drop of moisture out of sawdust. A bright light flashed in my face. It shut my eyes on a vision of Pepe looking closely at me. I heard short Spanish phrases. The motor revved up. There was the force of lift on my ankles, pressure down the back of my head. We were climbing. I tried to imagine I was somewhere else.

Climbing, then, I was back in Quebec, gently flying up the snow slope of Mount Saint-Laurent in a ski lift, drifting across the sunny wind, with the cool taste of pine in the air. And I could hear Valerie's happy laughter rising from the bottom of the hill. But all of a sudden I did the one thing they had warned me not to do. I looked down between my skis.

Next I was falling down an endless drop of vertigo to where Pepe and Jesus sat waiting for me. Back in Mallorca, in this ambulance on the road out of Soller, I was trapped.

"Then count the curves," I said to myself.

The Soller Pass is thirty-four curves up, twenty-eight down, a total of seventy-two hairpin bends in less than ten kilometers. I had crossed it many times in our red Mini on shopping trips to Palma from the mountain village of Fornalutx where I live with my wife and our two children. It means one hour of vigorous steering in nerve-wracking anticipation of a head-on crash with a bus full of tourists at every turn. Being the kind of nervous husband who does not trust his wife at the wheel, I usually insist on taking over for this stretch; so I know every turn in the road, precisely where to shift gear, when to blow the horn, and I can take in the scenery with my eyes shut. Up the mountain slope rise terrace above terrace of olive groves more ancient than Christ, they say, with gnarled old trunks piercing the stone walls in twisted poses of reclining growth. You wind your way up to the pass with the growing impression that the treetops will never make it to the level of the road. Clouds, when there are some, hang low over the curve you left behind a minute ago. There is an occasional pine, of the type that does not look at all happy in these surroundings.

But counting these curves was not like counting your sheep. "Where are you taking me?" I heard myself speak out at last.

"To Palma," said Jesus.

"But where in Palma?"

"To the hospital," said Pepe.

9

"Why?"

They said nothing.

"Please," I insisted.

"Shut up, Roberto."

"Sleep."

I tried. I wanted desperately to sleep. And perhaps I did for a while. I do not remember. That dull pain in my head is what I recall next. My face, too, began to hurt. And at the same time I could see Valerie, her long black hair flowing wild, her eyes frightened, pleading.

"Where is my wife?"

Jesus and Pepe exchanged a brief look.

"For God's sake," I pleaded. "Where is the senora?"

"Thy senora goes well," said Jesus.

"Sleep, Roberto," Pepe said.

"Does she know where I am?"

"La Senora is coming with her car," Jesus said. "Now shut up and sleep."

I felt better. And I must have drifted off on the image of the red Mini with Valerie at the wheel, speeding to my rescue in the night. We were riding flat and smooth. I could tell we had reached the Coll, that short stretch of level road between the climb and the descent, where Valerie and I usually stopped for a beer at Isidro's bar.

I now woke up fully, thinking that I had never been so thirsty in all my life. The first thing to do when we got to the hospital would be to ask for a glass of water, I decided. Perhaps Valerie herself would bring it to me.

But it wasn't Valerie's face that now flashed in my mind at the thought of drink. It was Rafael's, full of blood.

"What have I done?"

The hot light was back in Jesus's eyes. He nodded slowly at me in a way that meant, "Plenty."

"Tell me," I turned to Pepe. "Did I hurt Rafael badly?"

Pepe said, "Thou knowest nothing, Roberto. Now sleep."

I looked at Jesus.

"Thou art crazy," he said.

"Yes," I thought to myself, "I must be going crazy, to get drunk like that."

The pain in my head gave way to a heavy, pressing sort of fatigue as I tried to remember what I had done. Rafael's bloody nose and surprised look kept flashing through a jungle of arms and legs and shoulders and fists in a wild round of violence that heated the sap of murder to boiling in my veins. Then someone was holding my arms behind my back, while someone else hit me in the face. I struggled to hit back. I was sure I could floor them all if only they'd let go of my arms. I pulled and shoved and pushed to free my hands.

"Why art thou so angry?" Pepe said in my ear.

Jesus leaned forward. "All is now terminated, Roberto."

"Patience."

"Sleep."

That was when I began to feel sorry for myself. I remember asking for my wife. Again they assured me that she was coming behind us—which meant that I would be able to speak with her as soon as we got to the hospital, I figured. Then on that thought, and on the sensation that we were now winding down the curves on the Palma side of the Coll, I drifted into a comatose drowsiness that was not sleep, really, but the stupor-like trance which comes when the last fumes of gin sweep over the brains, leaving you with no lucidity

11

to control your emotions. Something hot and wet ran down my cheeks, and while one part of me would not surrender to such weakness, another side of me found a measure of soothing comfort in this release. The salt of tears soon began to sting, so that I realized I was wounded in the face. And this added a touch of pleasure to the self-pity. Precisely why I was crying, however, is hard to tell. I recall feeling miserably guilty. Not knowing exactly what terrible crime I had committed seemed to be the worst part of it. I knew I had struck Rafael and that perhaps he was badly hurt. There were others, too, who were at the Bar Centro when I got there and started swinging like a wild logger. But somehow I felt it was Valerie I had hurt most of all. And it was undoubtedly this haunting, bitter guilt which made me come to again, but in a fierce mood of fighting, this time.

"You brute!" I said to Jesus. "You have let me down."

He looked at Pepe, shrugging as if to say, "Here he goes again!"

I wanted to strike him. He and I had often met at the Cafe Santa Marta, and I had grown to like him in spite of the green uniform. He was courteous, soft-spoken, and I knew he could be kind. He had helped me to get back home one night a few months ago, after I had drunk till I could not make it alone up the mule steps from Santa Marta to Balitx. Afterwards I had thanked him with an autographed copy of my first novel. Maybe someday he would know English well enough to read it, he had said; in the meantime he was much honoured, though sad that this valuable present should come to him on the occasion of my having drunk so much.

"Why didn't you do like the last time?" I now said

to him. "You should have taken me home when you saw I was drunk."

"I was not there," Jesus said. "I was regarding the bulls at the Centro."

"That's a lie."

"Jesus does not tell lies," Pepe said. "It was *me* at Santa Marta."

"That's right!" I thought out loud, suddenly remembering. El Vitti was aiming for the kill on the small screen across the room, and Pepe was sitting two tables away with Marie-Noel leaning on his shoulder. A woman was drinking with me, when all of a sudden I found myself alone, feeling a great weight on my back and shoulders, and not wanting to leave here for a long, long time.

"Then why didn't *you* take me home?" I said to Pepe. "You must have known I was dead drunk?"

"But thou wert not intoxicated."

"What do you mean? God-dammit, I'm still drunk!"

"Thou art not well, Roberto."

"Thou hast written too much."

"Who says so?"

"The whole village knows it."

"Shut up, you liars."

It now seemed that we had been shouting at one another for a very, very long time. I could tell that all the curves of the Soller Pass were behind us. We were driving on the flat stretch leading into Palma.

"Christ, I feel drunk."

"Thou art not drunk. Thy head is a rare one."

"Thy brains hast performed a somersault."

"It comes to pass with artists, sometimes."

Then all of a sudden the cold rage took hold of me once again. I wanted to strike them shut. "Brutes!" I heard myself scream. "Liars! Let me free, then I'll show

13

you." I felt that I was going to choke. "Cowards."

"Shut up."

"Sleep."

"Bloody, shameless ones!" I went on, thrilled to be letting out the worst insult you can throw in the face of a guardia. Yet it wasn't enough. When drunk I can easily get a metaphor started, especially if it is to be used as a weapon. "You are nothing but the balls of Franco," I spat out. "And without you he's nothing but a dead prick."

"Roberto!" Pepe shouted. "Thou hast insulted Franco."

"Cojones!"

"Now thou hast insulted our body, our Cuerpo."

"Balls," I repeated. And with a two-word obscenity related to that same body I went on to tell them what they could do with their Cuerpo. The sound of my insults filled my ears. I loved it, savoring the recklessness of it as if I were on my tenth forbidden gin. Then I topped it all with what I thought must sound like a crushing, triumphant laughter of contempt.

What took place afterwards now seems even more vague than what I can remember up to the moment of my wild burst of laughter. The exchange of threats and insults must have continued for some time. I often have visions of scenes impossible to bear. But I will never know exactly what happened for the rest of the way. The Guardia Civil will not tell.

*   *   *

Jesus and Pepe had disappeared when I woke up again. I was now lying under a sky full of stars, and it was chilly. An old man with a bald head bent over me. "Poor senor," he said. "What has come to pass?"

"I feel tired," I told him. "Very tired."

14

"They will take good care of you in this location," he said kindly.

"Where am I?"

"Do not preoccupy yourself," he said. Then into the dark behind my head he whispered, "Regard his poor face."

"God of mine!" another man whispered back. "What have they done unto him?"

"Is there a small red car around here?" I said. "A foreign car."

"Do not worry," said the man with the bald head. "She will come, your senora."

They lifted me off the ground, gently, firmly. And it was strangely pleasant, this sensation of being carried across the night with your face up to the stars while steady footsteps on a gravel path sound near, travelling with you. Tall, narrow windows sailed slowly past on my right, then on my left I saw young blades of grass shooting out of a stone wall. It occurred to me that perhaps I was being taken through the garden of some ancient monastery converted into a luxury hospital for foreign residents of Mallorca. I heard the sound of keys. A high door opened ahead of us. We entered, turned right into a narrow corridor lined with high walls—whitewashed yesterday, I thought. In between bright spots of yellow light flashing from bare bulbs overhead I counted the beams as we moved along. But I could never get beyond ten, it seemed—the ten beams of our bedroom in Balitx?

Suddenly we turned left, then stopped. Again I heard the sound of keys. Another door opened. We passed a narrow doorway into a place that was well lit, then went on for several steps farther. I began to figure that this was a very large room indeed, when they finally put me down.

15

Four faces appeared abruptly out of nowhere, dark Spaniards crowding over me. They seemed surprised. One of them put out a hand towards my forehead; two of the others elbowed him not to touch. I asked what hospital this was. In reply they all set to work undoing the straps and lifting the blankets, not saying one word. They wore brown frocks and there was a mixture of concern and kindness in their eyes. Each one of them carried a set of large keys that fascinated me. Again I asked for my wife.

Two of the men bent down to help me to my feet. I waved them off, saying I would get up by myself, and at the same time I tried. Once on my elbows, however, I began to wonder if I could make it all the way up: my back would not bend from the sharp pain as I tried to sit, my hands and face were burning hot, my right knee felt as if locked forever.

I looked up at the four attendants. They stood there watching me with fixed, interested looks of gamblers who had just laid down their bets. I tried once again, biting tight against the pains.

Next I was standing in the center of a room the size of the plaza in Fornalutx. There were beds everywhere, and people in them. Not one head moved, however. But some of them must be aware by now that a new patient was being brought into the ward, I thought. It was hard to shake off the impression that they were all dead.

Why wasn't I given a private room? When would I see the senora?

The men looked at one another, shrugging that they did not know. Then one of them went away saying he would find out. The others closed in on me, gently urging that I undress and get into bed.

"That one, in the far corner."

Now, there are things I have a strong dislike for and will avoid at all costs. Sharing a taxi, eating with strangers, riding in a crowded bus or subway, using the stall urinals at train stations, are some of them. And it is the same with undressing in front of medical attendants, no doubt a throw back to my Air Force days and the humiliation I used to feel each time we were called on a "short-arm inspection" parade. Yet this time I took off my clothes without the slightest hesitation, in a mood of reckless fun, almost, as though watching my own performance in a crazy shadow dance.

The men in brown frocks smiled, nodding that I was being a good patient. They told me I could keep my underwear on. I said thank you. Then they escorted me to bed. One of them went through my pockets and found one hundred and twenty-seven pesetas, two packs of cigarettes, which he would give to the nun in charge of the ward, he said, to be returned to me in the morning. And now to sleep for a long, needed rest.

He had hardly finished speaking when I felt the cold touch of metal gripping my wrists. I looked to either side of the bed; two brown-frocked men were locking a pair of handcuffs on me. Each handcuff was attached to a large chain of the type we use to hang the pump at the bottom of our water cistern under Balitx.

"Please," I burst out. "Don't do that to me."

They tightened the handcuffs till I screamed from the pain.

"I have claustrophobia," I cried. "A bad case of it. Do you understand what I mean? How do you say it in Spanish, claustrophobia?"

The men looked at one another as if I had suddenly broken out into English. I tried to calm down and explain that I was going to choke to death if they chained me up. It was one of those weird diseases I

17

happened to suffer from, I told them.

They stood at the foot of the bed looking sorrowfully down the length of me.

"Take them off," I pleaded. "What kind of hospital is this? Take those chains off, for God's sake."

One of the men declared, "The gentleman finds himself here for judicial reasons."

"Have I killed anybody?"

"We do not know it. Our duty commands us."

"But why these chains?"

"It would be regrettable if you did harm unto yourself."

"Christ!" I thought, sinking.

The sound of footsteps in the corridor gave me a sudden lift. I was sure it was Valerie, at last. I tried to take a deep breath; it felt as if the chains were literally binding my chest. But this will pass, I told myself; Valerie will surely tell them about my claustrophobia and they will unlock the chains immediately. The important thing now was to remain calm, let her do the talking.

But it wasn't Valerie at the door. Instead I saw an old man dressed in a dark coat and wearing a soft hat. He came forward carrying a bottle and a wad of cotton wool, paused at the foot of the bed, exchanged a few words with the attendants, then stepping up to me he introduced himself as the night doctor.

"Would you please tell them to unlock these chains?" I asked him.

"Si, si," he spoke softly, almost in a whisper. "Later on."

"Now, please."

"First I must attend to your face," he said. "Do not move. Now, it does not hurt, does it?"

It did. But I did not mind. He was gentle with the

18

cotton wool, and that made up for the sting of
antiseptics burning the fresh wounds. He wanted to
know what had happened. I explained that I had drunk
and been in a fight. He then asked what kind of
foreigner I was. I told him I was born in Canada.

"English Canada?"

"French," I said. Most professional men in Mallorca
like to show off the little French they know, so I
switched to that language. "But I haven't lived in
Canada for many years."

"How long are you in Mallorca?"

"Four years."

"In Fornalutx?"

"Yes."

"And what do you do?"

"I write books."

He smiled. "And drink a little?"

"Sometimes, when the work goes bad."

"I understand," he nodded, then said, "So you do
not like these chains."

"Not at all."

"Will you promise to stay in bed, if—"

"I give you my word of honor."

He put out his hand. I shook it warmly. "Thank
you so much."

"Nothing," he smiled kindly. Then back in Spanish,
"May you get well."

As soon as he had walked away, the men in the
brown frocks undid the chains. Then one of them gave
me a pill and I drank two glasses of water with it. Once
more I asked about my wife. The senora was not here,
they said, but she would surely come in the morning.

"What time is it?" I asked.

"Past twelve in the night."

The men put out the lights, walked out and locked

the door from the outside. When their footsteps had died away, way down the other end of the corridor, I could still hear the sound of keys, faint now against the moans and snores and heavy breathing that filled the dark of the ward.

After a while the place began to smell like the pissotiere on the Soller Plaza. Somewhere in the night a woman shrieked. It sounded as if she was buried in a dungeon under my bed. Her screams stopped suddenly. In a moment I heard chains climbing up the metal legs of my neighbour's bed.

The fellow must be dreaming, I thought. Then longing for the effect of the pill, I drifted off, as the day began to dawn all over again in my aching, weary mind.

*   *   *

It had started like all the other writing days of this last month. I had gone up to my study early in the morning, spent a few hours on Manitou, then abruptly left the book feeling discouraged, miserable. I was bogged down on the fifth chapter of the novel. There were no writing problems to speak of; another ten or twelve pages only and that would mean the end of the first half of the book. Yet after many starts I could make no headway, today's effort yielding nothing more than a senseless rewrite of what I had rewritten yesterday morning and the morning before.

So I came down from my study and tried to keep busy with little chores around the house. I trained new shoots of the vine through the bower on our downstairs terrace, gave a second coat of green paint to a table in the nursery, then repaired the light switch in the washroom upstairs. But in the meantime I drank two gins in order to forget that I really ought to be writing instead of doing this kind of work. Naturally, I could not have been in a very pleasant mood when we sat down to lunch, so I promptly went through the first bottle of wine in the hope of cheering up a little, then feeling gloomier still I opened a second bottle and managed to empty it before the meal was over. The rest of the afternoon was spent arguing with Valerie. In the end we said very nasty things to each other and I had put away another three gins. The black mood was around the corner. I could sense it.

It was now five o'clock, time to watch the bull fight on television. El Vitti was in Madrid and I did not want to miss it. After telling Valerie I did not care to have her along, I left Balitx and walked down the mule steps towards the Bar Centro in the centre of the village. But when I got there and saw Rafael at a table near the bar, I decided to watch the fight somewhere else—in the last year or so I had carefully avoided finding myself in the same place with him. There was another cafe, the Deportivo across the plaza. But the place was full. Katie Schlicht sat on the terrace sipping a drink over a stack of postcards. I invited her to watch the fight at Santa Marta down the road.

"Delighted!" she said. But she had a few more cards to write, so would join me in five minutes.

"Fine!"

Then gradually, as I walked towards Santa Marta, thinking about Katie and her husband Theo and how much I liked them, I felt overcome with joy, happiness and sheer human warmth. It is always like that with me just before the onset of the black mood. The sombre, violent hatred is preceded by a great wave of brotherly love which leads me to buy drinks to strangers, embrace my enemies, melt into effusive sentimentality the spectacle of which would move people to swear I am a good drunk. It was in a similar spirit that three times

21

last winter I had treated Rafael to shots of Carlos Primero as a peace offer; he had accepted the drinks, but we had not shaken hands. Had I met him on the road to Santa Marta, presently, I probably would have done the same thing, and the evening might have taken a different turn.

Anyhow, at Santa Marta I bought drinks to Pierre and Therese, the owners, and had one with them. Then while waiting for Katie I had another drink with Juan, a Peninsular who was the brother of Manolo, one of Rafael's masons. We had asked him lately if he could get one of his sisters from the Peninsula to come to us as a maid. He had said yes at first, then no, and had not explained why. But as we touched glasses for the third time now he finally admitted that the whole thing had fallen through because, as Manolo's brother, he did not want to appear to be doing us a favour since Rafael might fire Manolo in retaliation.

"Sorry, senor Roberto," he said.

"I understand," I told Juan. "Thanks for trying, anyway." And I quickly took a long drink, then another one, to wash down this setback.

And I thought: goddam-it, a foreigner in Fornalutx needed only one enemy to turn the village against him. So I must come to terms with Rafael sooner or later if I was going to continue to live here with my family. This I had known for a long time. Only, how could I make peace with him and save my face when it was he who had done wrong and he wouldn't meet me halfway.

That was what I was trying to explain to Katie, next, sitting at a table in the back of the room, when all of a sudden I saw El Vitti enter the ring with the muleta. I had missed the early passes, the pics, the banderillas.

"Now I want to watch this," I said.

"Then stop ranting on against Rafael," Katie told me.

El Vitti worked superbly with the muleta. He could kill well, also, which was rare these days. I watched him go through a series of natural and aided passes, then round up with a perfect De Pecho in a slow, graceful and daring encounter that brought *Oles* from the stands and left the bull staring all around in dumb surprise while he calmly walked away with his back to the horns and, chin up, treated the crowd to that Manolette-profile pose which had become his trademark over the years. He obviously had a good bull, and there was a lot of fight left in him; so we were in for a fine kill, I thought. And I braced myself to watch it, straining hard against wave after wave of gin mist blowing across the screen. But after a while the ring went blurred, and El Vitti seemed to be coming in and out of focus. Or was it Jaime Ostos, now?

"Hey!" I shouted at Pierre to hurry up and fix that damned set. People in front of us turned and told me to keep quiet—"Please, senor Roberto!"

I remember feeling annoyed. Then I was telling myself that I had drunk too much, I must not finish this refill. There were bursts of *Oles* from Madrid, much shifting around in the room. And that, too, bothered me. I wanted to hear what Katie was saying in my ear.

She had been giving me a mild sermon on work, I believe. Hard work was the only thing that could sustain an artist and keep him from going around the bend, she said. But in order to work you must first rid yourself of the obsession that the whole world was against you simply because you happened to be different.

"Yes," I agreed. Artists were different. It was tough as hell to feel different all of the time, though.

23

"I understand," she said. So did her husband. Theo was chief psychiatrist in a mental hospital near London, so he knew only too well what could go wrong with artists. Did I know he was very fond of me, how much he admired my work?

"Well, that's fine," I said. And I, too, liked Theo. That was fine, fine. . . .

Suddenly, Katie was no longer there. I stared down the bottom of my glass, saw nothing but a shrinking slice of lemon. A tremendous weight pressed on the back of my head. I wanted desperately to lie down, but in order to lie down I must first get up from this chair, and that seemed to be the most difficult thing to achieve at this moment. Pierre must help me back home, I thought. He had done it before. He was a friend of mine. I must ask Pierre to take me home right away.

That was the last thought on my mind before the black mood struck.

*   *   *

Searching my memory for what had happened next, as I lay drifting in and out of sleep, I could find nothing but images flashing on and off across the night in the ward. And that is how I knew I was finally sobering up. It was always like this: a gradual, terrifying realisation that I had blacked out. Where I now was seemed less important somehow than the reasons why they had taken me here. So I must try and remember. . . .

But how can you recall what you were not conscious of doing at the time you did it? Even today, as I write this, I cannot recollect how I left Santa Marta, where I went from there, what I did up to that horrifying scene at the Centro. A real blackout it was indeed. It had happened to me before and I knew only too well how difficult it is to remember. All the guilt

24

and shame of unutterable disgraces will not pierce through those patches on the brains where drink has burnt the cells of consciousness to a gnawing atrophy. And the harder you try to remember, the worse it gets. Feelings of guilt and shame are the very stuff the blackout needs to tie up the ends of the vicious circle you cast around yourself on the carousel of drinking rounds. You desperately need to know what harm you may have done, but the guilt and the shame will not give you a chance to find out.

Sobering up then was crawling on all fours up the slimy walls of a nightmare pit. And to have known the feeling before did not help now. For that reason I made a strong effort to concentrate only on those images which had now begun to come back full, vivid, though disconnected. There would be plenty of time to find out about the rest later on, I thought. Then perhaps I had been lucky again and not caused too much damage after all. Besides, I had a hunch that some people in this place would want to ask a lot of questions before the brown-frocked men could let me out again. So I tried to place those flashes of recall in what I imagined might be their proper sequence.

First there was the bewildering montage of violence and blood at the Bar Centro, those same visions which had haunted me in the ambulance. But the only order I could impose upon them was that of cause and effect based on the supposition that it was I who had started the fight and was responsible for all that blood on Rafael's face. There was no other way to explain to myself the sight of two men holding my arms behind my back while three or four of the locals took turns swinging wild for my face. All right, I must have had it coming, I supposed. "So forget about that for now."

Then there was the jail in Fornalutx. I could see myself crawling on a stone floor in a cave. A pale light that must have come from the moon shimmered in through a small window near the ceiling. I saw bars, got up and leapt at the door, which I kicked, punched, and kicked, screaming at the top of my lungs to get me out of here, until the next thing I knew I was lying on the floor again, feeling cold and listening to the echo of my own moaning sounds. An avalanche of boots and trousers, leather belts and pistol holsters, came tumbling down upon me. I saw the chin of Jesus, the eyes of Pepe, the caps of other guardias. There was the Cabo's mouth nearly touching my forehead. I could not understand why he was so angry, why he must shout so loud simply to tell me that I was insane. Then I was up on my feet again screaming at them to leave me alone and send for a doctor.

It was cold. The walls were panels of sweaty cement. I urinated on the door.

The guardias came back after a while. With them was Theo. I tried to hit him, but missed. They took him away into the pale light. I lay back on the stone floor, shivering for I don't know how long.

Finally, there was the ride in the ambulance. Then all was black again, silent, still.

*   *   *

The noise of chains on metal woke me up again. I traced the sounds to a human shape rising out of a bed across the room. The chains dragged on the tiled floor for a few steps, then were heard no more. I held my breath. In a moment I could hear someone discreetly urinating in a tin bucket.

"Where the hell am I?"

Gradually, as I asked myself the same question a dozen times and over, the first light of dawn moved in

26

to make the rough contours of the place discernable. The wall on my right became three large windows, but set so high nobody could ever reach them, I thought, and each window was crisscrossed with iron bars. For a second I thought I was back in the jail of Fornalutx. But no! There was no escaping that I was sober now. Either this was the jail section of a hospital in Palma, or the hospital section of the Palma jail. "Take your choice."

So here I was in the hospital section of the Palma jail, I promptly decided. And the best way to face it was to dig into the reserve of delusions I had accumulated over the years.

I do not know how it works with other writers, but for my part I have found that a somersault of the imagination can come in handy at times, especially when the going is rough and you have run out of steam. If I was able to struggle for twelve years before seeing any of my work in print, it was thanks to constantly telling myself that repeated failures were essential to the making of any writer worth his salt. Also, I had read biographies of novelists and discovered that while I had little talent I had at least a lot in common with many of the writers I admired. Thus a headache of mine was not just an ordinary headache, but the same malaise which Dostoevsky suffered when he thought he might get another attack of the Grand Mal. If I had a bad row with my wife and my awful temper had been the cause of it, then I would think of Tolstoy and his bursts of thunderous wrath. When I had pains in my chest, they must be the same chest pains Balzac knew after drinking so much black coffee to maintain his schedule. The dressing gown I worked in on winter nights often warmed me up with the suggestion that I might have borrowed it from Flaubert himself. And

27

what a discovery when I read that Hemingway not only wrote longhand, as I did, but also used number-two pencils, the kind I always insisted on. In other words, my own failures seemed easier to bear when I could share some of the difficulties and idiosyncracies of great writers. Delusions of that sort cause no harm, I had always thought, while the escapades they inspire will often provide that extra pull in a rough passage.

And this time my imagination was quick to come to the rescue once again. "What the hell!" I now thought. "Norman Mailer spent two weeks in Bellevue after knifing his wife, and he's still a writer." And when this one began to pale I invoked the case of Tom Wolfe, that time he landed in hospital after a brawl at a tavern in Berlin—how many stitches in his skull? And still he had been able to write after that.

Dawn, meanwhile, finished dressing the barred windows with nispero leaves that now filtered a cool, greenish light into the room. I could hear the gay morning airs of birds outside these thick walls. I wondered what time it was, then realized my watch had disappeared. They would probably bring it back later on with the rest of my clothes, I reasoned. In the meantime I should remain calm and try to take in as much of the place as I could. After all, wasn't that what a writer ought to do in such a situation?

So I started by counting the beds. There were twenty-one—not including mine, of course. Then I counted twenty-one human shapes under the blankets, all of them tied to chains that were attached to the legs of the beds. Near the foot of every other bed were tin buckets in which to urinate, and to judge by the mess around them you could imagine how many of the patients had failed to aim properly during the night.

Next I tried to see what the people looked like. But

the few faces I could spot from my corner revealed no clues to what crime these men might have committed. Sleep gave them all a look of innocence. Now and again one of them would moan as in refusal to wake up yet. At one point I heard a loud, violent and insistent banging on doors somewhere up the corridor. Then came the sound of keys, followed by a short exchange in voices strained and low. Doors were unlocked, I heard a sudden, high whining cry, abruptly stilled and silenced, then the locking of doors again, and again that strange sound of keys.

The patient next to me had begun to move. He now turned and I saw that he was an old man. His head was shaved, he looked sleepily in my direction but did not seem at all surprised to find me here—which puzzled me, somehow. There was a vacant, lost expression in his eyes, a touch of kindness also, and I could not imagine that he might be so dangerous a criminal as to have to be chained. I was about to ask him what kind of prison or hospital this was, when he gave me a sweet smile, then turned the other way and went back to sleep.

A feeling of uneasiness crept over me. I had never been in prison before, but I could never have imagined that the atmosphere of a prison might be so weird as this. Even in Spain, I thought. And next I did not know what to think. I could hear strange noises as of chains being rattled very lightly, or discreetly tampered with, and I hurriedly scanned the beds anticipating that one of these twenty-one human shapes would suddenly leap up from under the blankets and dash for the doors— freedom at last! The rattling chains attracted my look to a bed along the wall, where a body was slowly hunching upon itself, with head lowered to nearly touching the pillow, and soon I made out the sad

29

spectacle of hands moving with steadily increasing speed under the blankets.

The fellow was still going at it a mile a minute, when the doors of the ward were flung open and four brown-frocked men walked in, to the clinking accompaniment of enormous keys. Three of the attendants went from bed to bed, unlocking handcuffs and waking up the men. The fourth came up to me.

"How do you find yourself?" he asked.

"I will feel much better when you tell me where I am."

"This is the Clinica Mental de Jesus."

"You mean, the Manicomio?" I said. "The nut house?"

"Si senor." He nodded, then added with a smile, "But do not worry yourself. We will take good care of you."

CHAPTER TWO

As a child in Quebec I heard a great deal about
asylums. In our family we regarded crazy people as
funny, insane people as dangerous; so we laughed at
the strange goings-on of the former but feared the sight
of the latter like the devil in person. We knew of course
that you simply could not be a Goulet if you were not a
bit touched in the head. But we never believed that the
Goulets were really insane. As our mother would put it
to us in her rare moments of tolerance towards our
father's parentage, we simply were a family of "nervous
ones." And whenever one of us behaved rather
strangely, why, he was merely being "not well,"
nothing more.

On my father's side of the family, four out of seven
great-aunts gave up the ghost inside asylums: Vinalda,
Sophia, Esmeralda and Lucinda. But when women had
such outlandish names and were old spinsters into the
bargain, the nut house must be the only place for them,
it seemed to us as children. Then there was Aunt
Yvonne, my father's sister, who drove her husband
Henri to the asylum and about whom my mother had a
very special way of speaking; she would never mention
her directly, but instead would refer to "Poor Henri"
with a long, mournful sigh, moving us to feelings of

pity for our uncle while our imaginations ran wild with a host of untold tortures Aunt Yvonne inflicted upon him. I remember her own terrible death as one of the earliest shocks of my youth. Her secret pleasure was to collect stray dogs, take them home, rub their anus with sandpaper, throw turpentine on the sore spot and then watch them writhe in pain while she recited the Rosary out loud for the alleged sins of her husband. But then one day, her current victim being of the larger breeds, the dog went knocking down the kerosene drum behind the kitchen stove and set the house on fire. Aunt Yvonne was then said to have atoned for her sins, roasting to death with beads in hand. And she had gone straight to heaven, where Uncle Henri would soon join her, we were told, for people who died in the asylum were innocent as babes in Limbo.

On my mother's side, the Roberts, two out of six uncles had to be put away fairly young. But as in the case of our father's family, we did not believe that Uncle Leon and Uncle Joseph were really insane. Besides, they themselves insisted they were at the asylum on vacation only, and we were told that they never mixed with the inmates. They used to spend one week with us each year; Uncle Leon was very good at knitting Argyle socks; Uncle Joseph could embroider pillowslips better than my sisters, and they always held each other by the hand when they had to go anywhere. One day I asked my mother what was wrong with our uncles, but was told to shut up, show respect for my elders, and that was that. Some years later I asked the same question again, and this time my mother turned a sad, worried look upon me, as if to say: "What is the matter, child, are you not well today?" I understood then that this sort of thing was not to be taken lightly.

And the impression has remained. Insanity had

cast upon me a weird spell of fear and fascination. I came to suspect that perhaps I carried in my blood more than a fair measure of ideas exclusive to the ones who are "not well." I even wondered at times by what unkind trick of fate I should have been given the names Robert and Goulet, considering how many "not wells" there were on both sides of the family. And I distinctly remember the sudden pause, an intimation of perjury, when I filled the questionnaire for an immigration visa into the United States several years ago: "Were you ever a member of the Communist party?" had been easy to answer, but "Is there insanity in your family?" had required a moment of painful hesitation before putting down a big NO.

Much later, as writing became less a matter of putting a book together than an obsession with driving a point of view to its ultimate clarity, I began to ask myself with increasing urgency if indeed there was not more madness than talent in my work. The more I wrote, the more solitary I grew. And the more I found myself alone, the more I wondered why I should so often feel that I was right and that everybody else was wrong. In other words, alienation seemed to become an essential part of writing. With time I grew accustomed to it, true enough. Yet the review of my first novel which bothered me the most was that one in Toronto which referred to me as "Pathologically angry. Mad!"

For at bottom I was terrified of such official identification. So long as I alone suspected that I was a bit mad, it was all right. I had made peace with myself on that score, anyway; which is to say that I had taken madness as one of my favourite subjects for jokes. Perhaps that was the better to master my fear of it, I do not know. At any rate, recurring doubts about my mental health had seemed easier to dispel if I could joke about it. I felt safe then, knowing I still had one foot on the outside.

*   *   *

But there was no joking about it this morning. I really was inside an asylum now. And I knew that I was cold sober, as I watched the inmates get out of bed and put on their clothes.

Indeed, how could I possibly be imagining such an extraordinary spectacle as this one? Not a word was spoken among the patients. They all moved very slowly, and with a concentration suggesting a private world accessible to nobody around, yet each man seemed to know exactly what the other man next to him was doing. It was like a perfectly executed pantomine, but with props, and if there was a silent director responsible for this odd performance, I could detect his presence only as a broad undercurrent of tenderness born of intermingling despairs.

The old man next to me now put on his trousers, socks and shoes, then another man from across the room came over to help him with his shirt. In return my neighbour bent down and tied the laces of the man who had just helped him. The two inmates then parted without a word, each one to tidy up his own bed.

There was a young patient in the far corner who had refused to get up after the brown-frocked attendant unlocked his handcuffs; instead he had begun to moan softly to himself, then to whine a little louder, as if the anguish that tormented him grew more painful with each minute that he was free from his chains. His lament now rose to such a pitch that I began to wonder why nobody seemed to hear it but myself. Then calmly, and exactly on cue, it seemed, another brown-frocked man made his entrance into the ward, walked over to

34

the screaming patient and slapped him across the face
with such violence that I was sure the poor fellow must
be unconscious, as he fell dead silent. Next the
attendant put out his hand, which the patient kissed in
a great burst of passionate gratitude. Then a short
while later the whole scene was repeated all over again.

Meanwhile the vague human shape that had
indulged in masturbation at the break of dawn finally
succeeded in stepping out of his pyjamas, and I now saw
the body of an adolescent, with the face of a very old
man, standing stark naked at the foot of the bed, penis
fully erect. One of the patients who had managed to get
dressed by himself and who obviously had the job of
cleaning the tin buckets, now stepped up to the lad
with mop and pail in hands, and whispered something
in his ear while gently tapping the erection down with
the handle of the mop. Next they kissed on the cheeks,
then the lad proceeded to put on his clothes while the
other went to work with the mop and the pail.

In the last few minutes I had noticed out of the
corner of my eye that a man on this side of the ward
was going through strange motions on his knees
between two beds. Turning my attention to him, I
gathered that he was saying Mass to some unseen
congregation somewhere in the wall, and on further
observation I made out a perfectly trimmed tonsure on
the back of his head.

A few beds beyond, a patient was folding and
unfolding his pyjamas. Next to him another one was
polishing his shoes most vigorously but with nothing in
his hands. My neighbour started knotting a non-
existing tie neatly around his neck. He smiled at me.

I smiled back, not knowing what to do, what to say.
He slowly leaned towards my bed. A feeling of
uneasiness bordering on fear came over me. He opened

his eyes very wide, as upon a discovery that fascinated him. Then suddenly he said, "Foreigner?"

"Yes," I sighed in guarded relief. "Canadian."

"Ah!" His eyes shot up to heaven, stayed there for a moment of intense search, then abruptly he smiled the polite grin of people who pretend to have just caught the punch line of your best joke, and with a slight bow of the head, he declared, "Welcome, senor Canada!"

"Thank you."

We shook hands.

"What are you doing in here?" I asked.

"Nothing."

"What is wrong with you?"

"I find myself very well in the head," he said. "But I am a nervous one."

"Been here long?"

"Twenty-seven years three months and fourteen days tonight," he reeled out in one breath. Then after a pause he hastened to add in a tone of strict confidence, "But I am leaving tomorrow. Tomorrow for sure—I mean, if my sister is willing." He looked all around as if afraid someone might be listening.

I took advantage of this pause to draw the attention of a brown-frocked man who had just entered the ward carrying a jug of water. He immediately came to the foot of my bed and asked what I wanted.

"My pants," I said.

"What for?"

"To urinate."

"Do you necessitate your pants to urinate?"

I did not know what to say to that.

"Senor?" he added, did I wish something else from him.

"Would you please bring my clothes," I said.

36

"Ah!" he grinned. "That is to say, you require *all* your clothes?"

"Yes."

"Good," he said. "I will tell the sister immediately."

As he left, I turned to my neighbour and said: "What's the matter with *him*?"

"He is a very good servant," said the old man. "Only, he has been here too long. Now there is something wrong with his head. But he is not a nervous one, though."

"No?"

"No."

"Cigarette?"

"Si."

"A match?"

"Forbidden. We must ask the servants."

"You call them servants?"

"Yes."

"Are they all like this one?"

"They are very good to us. You will see, after you have been here for a while—"

"But I am leaving this morning," I hastened to interrupt.

"Naturally. You and I will leave together, as a matter of fact. Now, what do they call you?"

"Roberto," I said.

"I am Jaime," he smiled. Then sitting at the foot of my bed, "Poor Roberto!" he said, "What has come to pass with you? Look at your face!"

In a few words I explained what had happened. He listened attentively, nodding gravely over the details of the fight. But when I mentioned Fornalutx, his old eyes lit up and I thought he was going to embrace me.

"Have you seen my oranges?" he asked. "I am of Soller."

"There are a lot of oranges in the Soller Valley."

"Si, si," he said, growing excited. "But my oranges, Roberto, they are not like the others! I created them myself. Listen, I travelled abroad, very far, all the way to Sevilla. From there I brought back some lovely ones with very delicate skin, with flesh so tender, so sweet. Then I took some Navels from the Valley, great robust Navels. And I put them together, like . . . like a quiet wedding in the shade along the foot of the mountains, over there, Biniaraitx way. You know where, Roberto?"

"Yes, I think I know where you mean."

"Then why have you not seen my lovely oranges?"

"I don't know, Jaime."

"They ripen very late in the spring, so they always sell themselves for a good price in Palma. We will be picking them very soon. You will come with me into the grove, Roberto, and I will give you an entire canasta for yourself." He paused, seemed lost in deep, sad thoughts for a while, smoking his nonlit cigarette. Then a long sigh flowed out of him and he said mournfully, "Ah, if only my sister had not become jealous, Roberto! If only. . ."

He would likely have gone on to tell me all about it, if we had not been interrupted at that moment by the arrival of the nun who was bringing my clothes. "Time for you to lay the tables," she said to Jaime.

He leaned forward and whispered to me. "You and I must take the four o'clock train to Soller this afternoon. Understood, Roberto?"

I nodded in agreement.

"Hurry up, Jaime," said the nun.

He asked her for a light. She pulled a Zippo out of somewhere in her skirts and lit his cigarette. He went away looking very happy with himself.

The nun dropped my clothes on the bed and said,

"Here you are, senor. You may get up now."

"Thank you," I said.

She was the nicest nun I had ever seen. And the most helpful, I thought, as the sight of my clothes moved me to nearly embracing her in a burst of gratitude. She looked fairly young, had a pleasant, cheerful face, and there was a note of authority in her voice that was not unfriendly. She gave me the cigarettes and pesetas found in my pockets. I asked if there was a message from my wife.

"Do not worry yourself," she said. "Your senora will come."

"You mean, she has not telephoned yet?"

"It is only eight o'clock."

"But—"

"Now you get up and put on your clothes. Then you will take some breakfast. Afterwards, later, you will see Don Guillermo. And after that, we shall see."

"Who is Don Guillermo?"

"The doctor in charge. He will examine you at ten o'clock. But you must eat, first."

"I am not hungry."

"Senor." She raised a forefinger in a gesture of mild scolding. "You must eat more, drink less."

"Yes."

"Someday you will say to me that Sor Catalina was right."

"Yes, Sor Catalina, yes," I said, somewhat impatiently.

She smiled warmly. "I will go and see if your senora has called," she said, and walked out of the ward, leaving me with the impression that we were great pals.

*　　*　　*

The only other patient left in the room was that old

39

man on his knees. And he was still folding and unfolding his pyjamas when I finally got out of bed.

Five or six faces appeared on both sides of the doorframe, staring at me like masks that had just been hung there to frighten me out of my wits. But they all looked more frightened than I was, suddenly, and one by one disappeared like puppets on strings.

"So here you are, Goulet; finally made it to the nut house, didn't you!" I thought to myself, as I started getting dressed. And I tried to imagine what my friends would say: things like, "Don't worry about it, this will give you something to write about." and "So what! It happens in the best of families."

But I derived little comfort from that, after a while. Nor could I find much consolation in the imagined company of great writers; to my knowledge the only one who had ever been inside an asylum was Nietzsche, and he had died in it. I thought about my great aunts, about Aunt Yvonne, about Uncle Leon and Uncle Joseph. But that did not help either. So there was nothing to do in the end but to repeat stoically to myself, "For God's sake, man, take it like a philosopher. Make the best of it."

Sor Catalina now came back. With her was a man in a white frock, whom she introduced as "Don Pedro, the practising one."

In one breath I said how do you do and when would I get out of here.

"Just a minute," Don Pedro said in a loud, cheerful voice. He gave me a friendly slap on the back. "Permit me to have a look." He examined my face. "How did *that* come to pass?"

"I got in a fight."

"But these wounds are not the result of blows."

"I don't remember."

"At best you rubbed your face against something."

"Maybe the floor of the jail," I shrugged.

"Well, that does nothing," he said. "It will all be cured in a few days if you do not pick at your face."

I said, "Can I get out of here right away?"

"Patience, Roberto," he said, dropping the senor as if he had been an intimate friend of mine for years. "I am only a male nurse. It all depends on Don Guillermo."

"What time is it?"

Sor Catalina looked at her watch and said, "Don Guillermo will arrive in one hour from now."

Don Pedro put one arm around my shoulders. "What is happening, amigo. Feeling depressed?"

I nodded yes.

"You drank too much last night. That is why."

"I don't like it in here," I protested, aware that he was scrutinizing me like some rare, valuable object, and that the nun also was doing the same thing. "You don't throw a man in a place like this just because he's drunk and got in a fight."

Don Pedro said, "Would you prefer the jail?"

"Yes."

"God of mine!" sighed the nun.

"Listen, Roberto," Don Pedro said. "Here in Mallorca we do this with any foreigner who gets excited. You are here for your own good. Do you understand? For your own protection."

It seemed to make sense. But I was in no mood to agree with them. "I still don't like the idea," I said. "A fellow will go crazy in no time in a place like this."

"Well, don't worry about that," said Don Pedro. "*You* are *not* crazy."

The way he said this made me wonder if he really meant it or if he was merely trying to appease me.

41

"You really think I *will* get out of here?" I hastened to ask.

"Roberto," he said with a shrug, as if I was letting him down. "Have patience, friend."

I said, "May I call my wife?"

"Your senora has telephoned," said Sor Catalina. "She will be here very shortly."

"Better, now?" Don Pedro asked.

"Yes," I said. "Thank you."

Then he said, "Why not give yourself a walk and look around the place? It's very interesting, you will see. There is a large garden outside. Take some fresh air. We will call you."

"But you must eat something, first," said Sor Catalina, walking out of the ward with Don Pedro. "Up there, at the end of the corridor."

*   *   *

For the first time since dawn I felt truly well. As I walked out of the ward my mind was clear, allowing my senses to know that I had pain in my back, that my right leg hurt above the knee and that my hands were hot and swollen. My face, too, awoke to a sizzling that lingered about the abrasions. And I welcomed this along with the other pains. Now that Valerie was on her way, I was sure to be released before noon.

Meanwhile I must try to make the best of my short stay here. "Why not take notes?" Think of it, to be locked up inside an asylum and yet be able to look at it from the outside! There was something to learn in this place, I thought.

I had hardly taken one step into the corridor, when a man approached me from behind and asked for a smoke in a low whisper you might expect between conspirators. I gave him a cigarette. He took it with fine, long fingers, shooting a short glance at me in a way that meant: "Don't look now, but I think we're being watched." He had a thin, long face and blond hair, unusual for a Mallorquine, and he wore an American-type raincoat buttoned up to the collar. The man reminded me of someone I had played tennis with in Quebec many years ago. I was beginning to wonder what could be wrong with him and how long he had been here, when he stepped up to me, casting furtive glances of alert up and down the corridor, and said in a whisper: "Just checked in?"

"Yes."

"How is the situation out there?"

"Fine, I suppose."

"Everything goes well?"

"I guess so."

He considered this for a moment, then stepping closer, so that I was forced to lean against the wall, he asked in a tense whisper, "What do they call you these days?"

"Robert Goulet."

"Robert Goulet?"

"That's right."

"French?"

"Canadian."

"Speak English?"

"Si."

He smiled, offered his hand and said in English, "How do you do. Good night."

"How do you do." I shook his hand. "Good morning."

"Are you well?"

"I'm fine, I think."

He thought for a second, then after quick looks all around, whispered, "This is a nut factory, you know," as if it were a secret only he and I had the right to possess.

"You think so?"

"You will become crazy in here. They will see to it."

I said nothing.

"Cigarette?"

I gave him another one.

"Thank you, Robert Goulet," he said with a wink. He lit up, gave me another "How do you do, good night," then hastily walked away, keeping close to the wall and carrying his head very low, as if bent upon a valuable secret.

Others must have seen me give him a cigarette, for the next second I was surrounded on all sides by nervous, wide-eyed inmates begging for a smoke. One full packet was gone before they would leave me alone. They all rushed to a brown-frocked man who happened to pass by: he pulled out his Zippo, shaking his head reproachfully at me. I continued on my way towards the dining room, thinking: "For God's sake, that's the least I can do for the poor wretches."

The corridor was long enough for a good stroll. And there were at least one hundred inmates walking up and down the length of it. Narrow, and with a very high ceiling, it nevertheless looked to me as if it might be as wide as the outside avenues of Palma, and I soon gathered that this impression was due mainly to the way the inmates walked: head bent, hands behind their backs, they rubbed against the walls rather than walked along them, and they cast side glances towards the middle now and again, suggesting a hundred private refusals to get involved in the traffic jam that wasn't there. So I had no choice but to keep to the middle of it myself, feeling increasingly self-conscious

44

as I went along. Everybody seemed most anxious to send a welcome nod my way, or a friendly smile. It was a most uncomfortable walk, and I remember telling myself something like, "I wonder if they feel as self-conscious as I do. After all, they must assume I am here for a look around only, that I am some sort of foreign visitor who has a special permission to visit the place. Unless ... unless they take me for one of them already!"

"But what the hell!" I promptly checked myself. "This is no way to be thinking, just before you face the psychiatrist."

So I shifted my gaze overhead in order to avoid all those eyes staring at me from everywhere. Full beams of bright morning sun poured in from large, barred windows on my left, but the windows were set so high you had the impression of being trapped in a whitewashed tunnel. At the end of it stood enormous doors, locked now.

Looking to the right, as I continued, I counted four large rooms like the one in which I had spent the night. I had a feeling that there were several floors above us, and perhaps other buildings somewhere outside. "Good God," I thought, "this is a large place!" And I wondered how many inmates it contained, how many were here for reasons other than mental illness. I wondered also if there were many violent cases among them. And then I wondered who among the ones walking behind me just now was going to jump on my back in a second. I turned round.

My conspirator friend of a moment ago was there, on my heels. He nearly bumped into me, his head down, shoulders hunched, hands in his pockets. And before I could recover from the weird discomfort of finding him next to me again, he whispered, "You are Robert Goulet," making it sound like a password.

I hastily gave him a cigarette, which surprised him as he had not asked for one. Then I hurried away from him.

What I really needed at this point was not food, but fresh air. One of the brown-frocked men had just unlocked the large doors at the end of the corridor. There was a rush towards the garden. I gladly joined in.

As we shuffled past the dining room, I saw my neighbour Jaime standing near the door with a tray in his hands. He spotted me, put the tray down on a table, and, raising one hand, sent me a "four o'clock" signal with fingers outstretched. I nodded yes, it was a deal, we would take the four o'clock train together to Soller this afternoon.

A little further on, just as we were about to step outside, I felt that someone was pulling at my right sleeve, and insistently so. Thinking it was my conspirator friend again, I pretended not to notice it. Someone on my left nudged me for a cigarette; I gave him one. Then I kept the packet in my hands anticipating that the man still tugging at my sleeve would want a cigarette also. But as soon as we had squeezed past the doors, he whispered in my ear, "Please, senor, can one speak with you for a second, if you permit?"

"Yes," I said. "What is it?"

"This way." He nodded to the right along the building, away from the other inmates. "If you wish to follow me, please."

I did, wondering what he wanted, what might suddenly flash from his dark, brooding look. He was short and had very broad shoulders that rolled faintly

46

as he walked. I thought that perhaps he had been a wrestler, or a prize fighter. After a few yards he stopped abruptly, grabbed my elbow and said with much feeling in his voice, "Welcome, senor. I desire to welcome you personally. I am proud of your wounds. You are one of us."

Not knowing what to say, I offered him a cigarette.

"No, thank you." He shook his head. "And by the way, it is worth more not to give away your cigarettes like that. They will never stop asking you. You will then terminate with none for yourself."

"I don't mind."

All of a sudden he grabbed my hands, pressed them warmly in his, and said, "Congratulations, senor. If it does not annoy you that I should say so, I estimate you as a man of honour. One of the night servants told me what you did. Congratulations!"

I shrugged that I did not know what he meant.

"How many guardias did you send to the hospital?"

"It was an unfortunate accident," I said.

"Oh!" His face dropped.

"I had had too much to drink and did not know what I was doing."

"Ah!" He seemed to cheer up again. "The same as for me. It always begins with one drink too many, then if one of those guardias comes around, he doesn't even have to open his dirty mouth, it is just the sight of them, I suppose, I do not know, but something happens in there." He tapped one side of his head with his knuckles. Every muscle in his face twisted. His hands became tight fists. Words failed him.

"You have got something against the Guardia Civil?" I said.

"It is a long, long story, senor," he sighed. "I have

47

dreams. Bad dreams. And they will not leave me in peace."

"How old are you?"

"I have accomplished forty," he said. "But I was not so young that I could not see everything and know what was coming to pass. They forced me to stand there and watch the entire massacre. It was my papa, then my mama, then my three big brothers, and then all of my four sisters, the total family. I remember how cold it was that morning. And the sun never dared to show up in the sky all of that day. There were black clouds, I remember, and they remained above us for many, many days. Then later, when I thought the sun might finally come out again, all I could see was an enormous winged cap hanging there above my head." Again he knocked on his temples, and his face became twisted. It was a while before he could go on. "It is those dreams, senor," he moaned. "Those bad dreams. They have been chasing me everywhere I go. There was Sevilla, Barcelona, then this place here five years ago. Then there was Barcelona once more, and now this place again, six months next week. I tell you truly, senor; there are not many manicomios in Spain where I have not been at one time or another. And it is always the same story. First come the bad dreams, then I take a drink to chase the dreams away, but as they do not leave me in peace I take another drink, and that makes it worse, the dreams just go on haunting me, until I take another drink too many, and by that time it is too late: one of those winged caps is sure to pop up, and I charge him like a brave bull."

"Cigarette?"

"Thank you." He took one, put it in his pocket.

I said, "Does it help you to be in a place like this?"

"Yes, it does. But for a little time only. I take the

48

electric shocks, you know. Don Guillermo says electricity burns bad dreams away and then I am supposed to find myself well for a while." He stepped up very close to me, looked all around as if we were being watched, then whispered in secret, "But you know what?"

"What?"

"There are dreams they cannot burn away."

"I suppose so."

"And you know why?"

"Why?"

"Because there are dreams people will not part with, ever," he declared with a knowing wink. "Doctors in all the manicomios have a name for my illness. But they are wrong. It is I who know, because—" He once again looked around in case anyone was watching or listening, then whispered very low in my ear, "Because I am not crazy; that is why. My problem is to have been born with a heart in my chest. I am a man of honour. There are many like me all over Spain, people who do not want to forget. So I must live with my bad dreams, no matter what comes to pass, no matter how many guardias it costs." He paused. "See you later, senor, Adios, amigo!" Then he quickly walked away, his broad shoulders rolling, his face proudly held up to the blinding sun.

*　　*　　*

Deeply moved by what I had just heard, I stood against the wall feeling sad, depressed, yet mellow with ancient longings. It felt as if I had just been told a few home truths about my own self perhaps long forgotten. There was nothing really new to be learned from the story of this poor fellow, I thought, only something old to remember, the way you recall an early act of faith, pure and passionate, or your first love, or again all the

49

dreams you had mortgaged to the claims of so-called growing up. What he had said about heart and honour now made me think about my work. I felt even more melancholy.

"But hell, I must get out of this mood," I promptly told myself. "It won't do to get depressed just before facing the psychiatrist. Got to cheer up, somehow. Make the best of this. Look around. Take notes."

The garden spread before my eyes like a set for some outlandish show I had not bought a ticket to. There were at least a thousand men walking up and down narrow paths and alleys that crossed and curved and crisscrossed in a maze of private strolls to nowhere. The walls that contained it all were as thick as those of Balitx, at least one full metre, and they rose so high you could see only the tops of the plane trees on the other side. Overhead was a flat expanse of sunny blue sky, yet more than half the garden lay still in the shade because of the high walls. And in the shade most of the men remained, carrying their heads down, their hands behind their backs, as they walked on and on, back and forth, each to his own secret destination, in silence. There was a look of determination about the way they walked, but not once did they run into one another. You could tell there would never be a collision here.

Then once again, as I had thought on first waking up in the ward, I had the strange impression that perhaps this was some sort of mad spectacle being put on for my benefit alone, so incredible did it seem that so many people should be locked up in one place and yet not clash with one another. In the center of the garden, where the sun poured a hot blinding light, an old man was crawling on all fours, with his nose almost to the ground, and I thought he was looking for cigarette butts until I realized he was merely trying to draw a perfect circle, looking back now and again like a dog to see if his tail was behind him. Then repeatedly crossing the old man's circle, dead centre now from one direction, then from another, came a bushy-haired lad who was either chasing after something on the ground or being haunted by something on his heels. Not once did the lad and the old man get in each other's way. Nor did they seem to mind that the path of one should cross the path of the other. It was as if insanity enabled them to mingle in perfect harmony.

And I wondered why it should be so, why there should be such a note of gentleness about these people, tenderness, even. Was it due to the fact that each man was locked up inside himself? How could a thousand private despairs produce such a peaceful intermingling?

Indeed there was great peace within these walls, a sense of security I had seldom known on the outside. I knew that I did not want to stay here one hour more, yet there was something weirdly inviting about the place. It had an order of its own, an impression of working out well, somehow, a quiet power of the kind that comes from things organized, smooth and lasting. And it all came about independently of any effort from your part, which was perhaps the secret of its strange appeal. It was good to sense that there was nothing to create, here, no problems to solve on your own, no order to impose out of your own guts. I found myself almost liking the place. There is no chaos in insanity.

Then all of a sudden Don Pedro was standing before me. "Come, amigo," he said kindly. "Don Guillermo is here."

CHAPTER THREE

So I must now prove that I was not insane! I had finally come up against a psychiatrist.

To me, a psychiatrist had always been rather like a country priest, a simple sort of fellow who honestly believed in what he peddled around but who really did not know what he was doing, yet one who managed to help people now and again. They earned a comfortable living at it, both of them, and neither one nor the other was truly dangerous or harmful, unless you happened to cross their paths at High Noon and with a different credo from their own.

Now, on the level of basic differentiation between myself and the psychiatrist, I had tended to regard our respective minds as bearing those polar distinctions which Pascal studied in "La difference entre l'esprit de geometrie et l'esprit de finesse." The psychiatrist's way of looking at things belonged to the former, mine to the latter, and although our basic preoccupations were compatible in that we both focussed upon the human condition, there nevertheless remained this difference between us: his approach was scientific, mine was essentially intuitive. The stuff of writing is a private soul of imagined truths glimpsed in sincere moods of feeling touched with awe. Until these fragile glimpses are given form, and even after, one is loath to expose them to scientific scrutiny, lest they become blurred or distorted by analysis or identification. To create is to clarify, and all the formulas of psychiatry will not yield one single living, moving clarification of the kind which goes into the making of a character in a novel. In that sense the psychiatrist is the writer's worst enemy, just as the writer, by the elusive quality of his knowledge, can become an intractable subject to the psychiatrist and, as a result, his worst enemy also. For that reason I had always kept my distance, feeling that we could not come together except for a duel of irreconcilable disciplines.

Which is not to say that I had refused myself all contact with psychiatry, however. As a drama student at Yale after the war, I had dabbled in a potpourri of Freud and Horney and Jung, as it was then claimed that you could not write without at least a working knowledge of analytical therapy. But I had soon found the whole thing irrelevant to what I felt writing was about. And from then on I had avoided the matter both in my reading and in my writing, content to retain from my contact with it only a passing knowledge of psychiatric terminology.

And that was all I had to fence with, I now realised, as I entered a small room half the size of my study—blinding whitewashed walls, a crucifix, a bare desk, a chair, then Don Guillermo greeting me with a pleasant smile. He motioned me to the chair. But he himself remained standing, telling Don Pedro to schedule a shock treatment for midday as an outpatient had just come in from Inca.

Don Guillermo was very short, and I wondered if he was remaining on his feet in order to overcome the psychological disadvantage of having to look up to me when I entered the room. His eyes were black, there

53

was kindness in them, a quick intelligence also, and they inspired confidence. On my guard, however, I immediately decided not to trust him: he seemed too friendly.

"Well, Don Roberto, what have you got there?" he said kindly, when Don Pedro had left the room. Then sitting down he gazed at the wounds on my face the way you study the little scratches on the hand of a child who has just hurt himself and must be humoured out of a crying fit of self-pity.

I offered him a cigarette. He declined with a smile. I took one and lit up.

Then I began to tell him briefly what had happened, that is to say, as much as I could remember.

His eyes would not leave my face while I spoke. Nor would they meet my look squarely. They slowly wandered all over my forehead and chin and nose and cheeks in that sort of gaze you use on people you set out to master into uneasy self-consciousness. And it worked, for I soon felt the heat of shame on my temples, and when I looked down at my hands and found them hideously swollen I felt a pang of guilt rather than pain. My blood circulation must have been affected, too, for my skin began to feel hot all over, and I sensed that it was not aching from the pressure of a thousand drops of alcohol sweating through my pores; no, I was getting angry, I could tell. So in the back of my mind I kept reminding myself to stay calm, not get excited. But that did not work. Before I could reach the end of my brief summary I abruptly broke off and asked resentfully, "But haven't you got a report from the Guardia?"

"Continue," he said.

"I can't."

"Why?"

"I don't know."

"Depressed?"

"Who wouldn't be, waking up in a place like this?"

He nodded that he understood.

"It isn't particularly cheerful in here, you know."

Don Guillermo pulled the middle drawer of his desk and took out a slim folder which he slowly opened and then set down between us. I saw my name in blocked letters at the top of a long sheet full of little squares. In a moment he began putting check marks opposite words and phrases that looked like questions to me. And I felt as if every cell in my brain were being reported upon after careful weighing and measuring. There was a chilling impersonality about it that frightened me even more than some of the anguished, obsessive and haunted looks I had seen on the faces around here this morning. And it got worse, as Don Guillermo continued to fill those little boxes with check marks, slowly, carefully and as if at the end of laborious consideration, asking me all sorts of questions at the same time. But who I was, where I came from, was I married, where did I live, and all of that, seemed to have nothing to do with those check marks he was putting down. He wasn't even writing down my answers.

"How do you spell your name?" he asked, when I told him I was a writer.

It was there. Both of us could see it. There was no need to ask me. Yet I heard myself spelling it slowly and with sudden joy: "G-O-U-L-E-T." I had never thought that the mere spelling of your own name could give so much comfort. I began to feel better, relax a little.

But that did not last long. Don Guillermo soon went on to question me about my work, a subject I

55

could seldom discuss without feeling ill at ease and resentful. Had I been published?

"Yes."

"What do you write?"

"Novels."

"How many are printed in book form?"

"One."

"Only one?"

"Well!" I had struggled for twelve years and written four novels before getting this one accepted; I had never felt in a hurry. But why tell him that? I thought. And I said, "Isn't one enough, for now?"

He smiled. "If it is good."

"It is an honest book," I said.

"Would you tell me what it is about, if it does not annoy you?"

Yes, I did mind. But again why tell him that? I thought. I had been asked that same question a thousand times before and had never been able to answer it. So I said, "It is about Canada."

"How interesting!" He looked up from the sheet of little squares on his desk. "Can one read it in Spanish translation?"

"It is not the kind of novel that is permitted in this country."

"And why?"

"The Catholic Church doesn't like it."

"So it is against the Church?"

"No. It is an honest novel, that's all."

He seemed puzzled for a second. Then a faint smile crossed his lips—a smile of amusement, I thought. Once again I had to tell myself not to get angry.

He said, "Is it a novel of protest?"

"Every honest novel is a protest," I said.

"Really!"

"In a sense, yes."

"So a novel of protest is an act of violence?"

"I wouldn't put it quite that way," I said. "I rather see it as the ultimate expression of a violent thought."

Resting his elbows on the edge of the desk, Don Guillermo leaned forward. "Now, according to what you say, there is no difference between a violent thought and a violent act?"

I felt a pang of panic. The conclusion was inescapable. I was trapped. Worse still, I could tell that he sensed it.

"I mean, strictly speaking," he drove on. "Are they not one and the same thing?"

"What?" I pretended to have lost my train of thought.

"A violent thought and a violent act," he pressed on, "are they not equal, according to what you said?"

There was nothing to do but give in, if only for a breathing spell. "Yes," I said. "Essentially, I suppose they are one and the same thing. But—"

"Now, about that man called Rafael," he interrupted, abruptly shifting back to Fornalutx and landing on the exact spot where I had left off in my summary. "You say you struck him in the face with your fist?"

"That's right."

"How many times did you strike him?"

"I cannot remember."

"Do you recall hitting him at all?"

"No."

"Then why do you say that you hit him?"

"I have that vision of him, with his face full of blood, so I assume I must have hit him."

"What you mean is, you intended to hit him?"

"Last night?"

57

"No. In the past, I mean, you intended to hit him in the past, did you not?"

"Yes."

"Now, did he provoke you last night?"

"Not that I remember."

"Did he ever provoke you at all?"

"Oh yes. Several times."

"Why?"

"He was jealous. I once had a maid he had been engaged to, and he claimed that I was going to bed with her. Oh, it's a long story!"

"One of those small-town intrigues?"

"That's right. The man became absolutely pathological about it. Made my life impossible. Threats here, insults there. He just wouldn't let off."

"Is he violent?"

"Runs his men with an iron fist. He threatened the mayor last year and they put him in jail, but he got out after two days. He was a fallangista, I hear. Used to belong to a firing squad—"

Don Guillermo cut me short by clearing his throat very loud, so that I knew I had stepped on forbidden ground. Then he said, "What I desire to know is: what do you think of this Rafael?"

I said, "What do you mean?"

"Do you feel any hatred for him?"

"I don't really know. Sometimes I feel sorry for him and I wish we weren't enemies. But there are times when I truly hate him."

"Why?"

"Let me put it this way. I don't believe I really hate him as a person, as an individual, that is. Rather it is the evil in him that I hate."

"Naturally," said Don Guillermo. "That is the writer's way of looking at it."

58

"Well, I am a writer."

"But what I mean is, there is also another way of looking at it. *Our* way. And in these circumstances it is our way that must prevail."

I offered him a cigarette. He refused it. I took one and hastened to light up.

"Isolating the motive behind the act is one thing," he went on. "And that is where *your* enquiry usually ends. I mean, you as a writer desire to know no more than just that. Yet there is a great deal more to it, you know. Here, we must also concern ourselves with remedies, therapy. For that reason we must seek to isolate the primary causes, what I desire to refer to as those dark secret obsessions which haunt people and sometimes drive them to acts of aggression." He paused, looked me straight in the eye, then said, "Fear, for instance?"

"Yes," I nodded. I could tell what he was driving at. Let him have the last word, I told myself. And I said to him, "Yes, fear can be deadly."

"Man always hates what he fears."

"That's right."

"Hate is a negative passion you promote in your heart in order to enable yourself to destroy what you fear."

"Yes," I agreed again.

"Then if you are logical, you must confess in the end that you are afraid of this man Rafael." He smiled. "Is that not the problem, at bottom?"

Now the slimy bastard is trying to tell me I'm a coward, I thought. And I said, "But as I told you, it is the evil in him I am afraid of, not the man."

He picked up his pencil. "Senor Roberto," he said. "I think you desire to fence with words."

"Isn't that what usually takes place when writer and psychiatrist meet?"

"I cannot know about that," he said sharply. "You are the first writer I ever interviewed as a patient." He began writing on a separate sheet of paper. After a few lines, he asked, "Do you feel sorry for what happened?"

I thought for a moment, then said, "Yes, I am sorry for the trouble I caused my wife."

"Is that all?"

"In the main, yes."

"But what about this man you hurt so badly?"

"I cannot remember actually hitting him. So how can I regret an action I was not conscious of doing at the time I did it?"

"You might have killed him."

"Did I?"

"I cannot know about that. The only thing we have is a verbal report from the guardias who brought you here last night."

"If he were dead, we certainly would know about it by now. No?"

"Most likely," he said, continuing to write what seemed to me to have nothing to do with what we were talking about. He did not pause to wait for my answers. Instead he just went on rapidly setting down what must be his own verdict, based on what I had told him about Rafael, I thought.

And I said: "Do you suppose I will be allowed to leave here this morning?"

"That does not depend on me," he said. And without a pause he asked again, "So, you do not feel sorry?"

"I wish I could tell you that I do," I said. "But in all honesty I don't feel sorry at all about Rafael, which

60

doesn't mean that I do not feel guilty, though."

"Very interesting."

There was a gentle knock at the door behind Don Guillermo's desk. He said, "Come in." I expected the sound of keys. I saw the door open slowly and without noise. A nun appeared and whispered, "Now," then disappeared.

Don Guillermo said to me, "You are now going to meet Don Juan, the director of the hospital. He is the person who has to decide. According to me, there is no objection to your immediate release. I find you in good health, though slightly obsessive. But I strongly advise you to stop drinking altogether, for a while at least. Another thing," he smiled; "it appears to me that you are a bit apprehensive about members of our profession. Someday you may have to learn to co-operate with us. Naturally, I take into account that you are not in the best of forms this morning."

"I am sorry if I was discourteous," I hastened to put in.

"I understand," he said. "If later on you desire to come to talk with me, do not hesitate. I should be delighted to see you again. Esta en su casa."

I stood up at the sound of approaching footsteps. So did Don Guillermo, just in time to greet his superior at the door. The two men shook hands. Then Don Juan walked up to me.

"So here is the Canadian with the bad temper!" He slapped me on the back. "How do you find yourself?"

"Fine," I lied.

Don Juan was as short as Don Guillermo, his face was marked with eczema, he wore thick glasses that magnified his eyes to a haunting look. Something bothered me about that look. I felt more uneasy than with any of the inmates I had met this morning.

"So you beat up a Mallorquine?" he said, as if it were a monumental joke.

"I suppose so. I cannot remember everything."

He laughed. Then turning to Don Guillermo, "And he insulted Franco into the bargain!"

Don Guillermo smiled.

"Anyway," said the director. "Do not worry about it for now. We will do the best we can for you while you are here."

"When can I get out?"

"Do not think about that," he said. "It will only make you more nervous. Try and enjoy your stay with us." Then abruptly dead serious, he turned again to Don Guillermo. "Your diagnosis?" he asked in Mallorquine.

"Very interesting," Don Guillermo replied in Mallorquine, and pressed a button on the wall. "I would like to keep him here for a while."

I felt a rush of blood down my legs, and had to sit down. But I did not care to listen to what they were now saying, still speaking in Mallorquine on the assumption that I could not understand. I could not believe that they really meant to keep me here. Nor could I believe my eyes—both Don Guillermo and Don Juan wore high heels!

In a moment I heard the sound of keys, then saw Don Pedro enter. There was an exchange of looks, which seemed to me to confirm my sentence. Don Pedro then put one arm around my shoulders and helped me up to my feet.

"Now, now, Roberto, don't you worry yourself," he said. "Your senora will be here promptly, and everything will terminate well. Come along, friend. You've had a rough night."

*   *   *

In the corridor were two lines of inmates facing one

62

another like sentinels at attention. Shaken up as I was, I thought for a second that this was a mass show of welcome in my honour, and expected them to salute, as Don Pedro and I marched between the lines. Was this the customary routing of initiation? Was I now being officially received as one of them?

"What's this?" I asked Don Pedro.

In reply he shoved me to one side, then quickly joined me and we stood in line with the inmates. "Do not move yourself," he whispered. "Do as we all do. Watch!"

I saw a tall, slim man with the face of a Don Quixote and the proud, dignified bearing of a Richelieu, walking towards us in the slow ceremonial pace of a monarch receiving his court. The men bowed low as he passed, some dropped to their knees, others crossed themselves. He paused to draw the sign of benediction over a prostrate head, or stopped to allow an old man to kiss his hand, while a low whisper of respectful greetings rose up to him from left and right.

Again I asked Don Pedro, "What's going on?"

"His Holiness," he whispered. "Pope Arturo the First." And he bowed.

His Holiness paused in front of me, threw his head back with an air of demanding to know why I should not be bowing to him as all the others did, then he gave me such a fierce look that I thought he was going to strike me in the face. Involuntarily I stepped back against the wall. A snorting sound came out of his pointed nose. Then he went on his way to the accompaniment of greetings from everybody: "Good morning, His Holiness! Please, His Holiness! A momentito, His Holiness, please."

After a few more steps, near Don Guillermo's door, Pope Arturo the First stopped short, slowly turned

63

instead of staying in the middle. A brown-frocked man came by.

"What time is it?" I asked him.

He pulled his watch from under his frock, looked at it and said in a lightly singing voice, "Eleven o'clock."

"Thank you."

Then back in the line of inmates walking along the wall, I thought, Good God! Valerie will never come. It only takes one hour from Fornalutx to Palma, and it's now more than two hours ago that Don Pedro told me she had left. Something must have happened. Maybe she is so upset she cannot drive the car. She has had an accident, maybe. Or maybe she doesn't know where I am. But that cannot be! She has telephoned already, so she must know I am here. Or maybe she hasn't called at all and Don Pedro says she will come because he wants to humour me out of depression. Pretend a little? Yes, so he is giving me the full treatment now! Or am I really going around the bend?

"Stop thinking," I told myself. "Look around. Stop thinking."

Looking around, I noticed an old man ahead trying to draw my attention by stepping out of line at every five or six steps, then looking back over his shoulder for a wink and a nod my way. He seemed harmless enough, so I quickened my pace and soon caught up with him.

"What is it?" I said.

He beamed with secret thrill. "Look down here." He lowered his eyes on his chest, his hands went under his jacket and he hunched his shoulders to protect what was there from the gaze of others.

"What have you got?" I asked him.

He quickly took it out and placed it in my hands, looking all around to make sure nobody was spying on

66

us. Then hunching his shoulders even more, he leaned over me for added secrecy.

It was a magazine. Spanish. The cover showed a torero and a bull at the moment of the death thrust. It looked like an old publication. I began to open it. But quickly the old man pulled it out of my hands, and his face broke out in an expression of deep sadness, as if he meant that while I could admire the cover I had no right to see what was inside. I had had time to catch the date, however, July, 1924.

"How long have you been here?" I asked him.

He stuffed the magazine under his jacket and whispered in my ear, "Since July, 1924."

That's a long time, I thought, forty-one years altogether. But then, July, 1924 was also the month I was born. "Good God!" I hurried away from him as from a bird of ill omen.

"What time is it?" I asked a brown-frocked man passing by just then.

He sighed, so that it occurred to me that this was the same attendant who had told me the time a moment before. I wanted to say, "All right, forget it." But he had already pulled his watch from under his frock. "Eleven fifteen," he said impatiently.

I thanked him. Then frantic to find something to do, or something to observe, so as not to be alone with my thoughts, I decided to enter the first door on the right.

Here was the bath-and-shower room. Not since my Air Force days twenty years before had I ever come across so large a group of men all naked in the same room. A shroud of steam gave a muted note of distance to the sounds they made while trying to wash themselves. I felt as if I were spying upon a playground of children in forbidden games on a misty dawn. There

67

must have been hundreds of them, and, naked, they all
looked alike. Indeed the only way I could tell the young
from the old was by the movements they made: how
quickly they jumped in and out of the tubs lined up
across the room like rows of graves in military
cemeteries, or how long they took to soak themselves
under the nozzles jutting out of the walls around the
room. They all seemed to be having a good time,
however, and the only ones who looked worried were
the few who had erections and just walked aimlessly
through the steam with an air of not knowing what to
do next. The traffic cops of the asylum, those brown-
frocked men with stern faces and dangling sets of keys,
wandered among them, now helping with soap and
towels, now shouting to hurry up—it would soon be
time for lunch; while two nuns on my side of the room
got busy distributing bundles of clean clothes to the
men as they came out of the steam shivering, self-
conscious in their naked states.

As I looked at them, I now came to think of all the
things they were not allowed to wear or carry on their
persons; no belt, no tie, no shoe laces, no matches, no
razor, no watch, no comb, no pencil or pen, nothing
sharp or hard, nothing they might try to kill
themselves or others with. They had their skin, and
that was about the whole of it. Or could it be that it
was their skin that bothered me so, as I looked on?
Young and old alike had that white sort of dry skin you
find on a fish that has lost its scales and been left to rot
in the sun. The flesh looked soft and saggy, so that you
sensed that it must smell, even when clean, and it
seemed to me that if you poked that skin there would
come no surge back nor bruises, for there were no
muscles left, not the least suggestion of quivering
nerves. Then it began to dawn upon me that the worst

who wandered in and out with bored looks and flat feet dragging.

Quietly, I went to a table towards the end of the room and sat with my feet on the bench. Then once again I tried to divide nine hundred by twenty, to find out when my next interview with Don Guillermo would come up in the event Valerie failed to get me out of here.

After a while I grew aware that someone was next to me. He had come silently sliding along the table to where I sat. And I welcomed him, for it was high time to start thinking of something else again, as I had just come to the upsetting conclusion that if I were to stay here I would see the doctor only once a year.

"Good morning," I said.

His greeting was a gentle smile, very different from the nervous, secretive way the others had approached me throughout the morning. And he offered me a cigarette, which I accepted. He must have been at least fifty, had a lot of white hair, the skin on his cheeks was still young, there were deep, vertical furrows above the bridge of his nose, and when he lit my cigarette I saw that his hands were fine and delicate. He wore a suit, with shirt and tie, and had a watch.

"What time is it?" I asked him.

He put out his wrist for me to see. It was twenty to twelve.

I said: "Are you a patient here?"

"That is to say, I live here," he replied, speaking in a soft voice that did not have any of the anguish I had noticed in the others. "But in the other wing," he added. Then in a perfect Spanish very little touched with the Mallorquine accent, he went on to explain that beyond this room was another department of the Clinica Mental where about two hundred men lived in

71

conditions considerably better than in this section.

"You do seem to have special privileges," I said.

"Naturally, as one pays one hundred and twenty-five pesetas a day. The food also is much better than in this section. Then we have private rooms. And as you can see, we are permitted matches and many of the things that are prohibited for the others in here. Naturally, one must consider that we are not so very ill, in my section. In fact, many of us are not ill at all."

I had a second look at him, as he went on, and it suddenly struck me that he did in fact seem quite normal. His eyes did not have that intermittent glossy stare of the lost mind I had seen in all of the others. There was something alive and constant about his look. Then as he talked I gradually began to feel that I was no longer within these walls. "Why, this man is just as sane as I am!" I thought.

"I have been here seventeen years," he was saying. "But I have managed to remain as healthy as when they first put me in. Not that they did not try to make me lose my mind. Besides, they really do not have to try very hard: the very circumstance of finding oneself here, surrounded with so much misery. . . Ah, Senor Roberto, if you only knew! It does not disturb you if I call you by your first name, does it?"

"Go ahead," I said. "What do they call you?"

"Ernesto."

"Glad to meet you, Ernesto."

He sat closer to me. "You see, Sor Catalina told me all that came to pass with you. So I had much illusion to meet you, especially as you are a writer. I read a great deal, but have never met a writer in person."

I began to feel ill at ease. "May I have another cigarette?" I said.

"With much pleasure." He gave me one and struck a match. "What do you write?"

"Novels."

"Ah! The stories I could tell you about this place! What a book it would make!"

"There is one thing I would like to know," I said. "How did you manage to spend seventeen years in here and not go around the bend?"

"Well, that is very simple," he said. "First of all, I was perfectly well when they locked me up, just as well as I am today. I was not vulnerable, as you might say, I was not already suffering from a mental defect. Then, rather than brooding over the injustice they had done to me, I used my mind to create something. I decided to become an inventor."

"Why did they put you here in the first place?"

He leaned over my shoulders. "I knew too much," he whispered. "It was this way, you see. I was the treasurer of a Medical Insurance Group in Palma, there came a scandal about the contributions, and I was very familiar with all the sordid details, so they simply had to put me away, in order to protect the higher-ups."

"I see."

"But I am not bitter," he hastened on. "Bitterness would have made me go completely insane in a place like this. So, as I said, I decided to become an inventor. It was only natural, I suppose; figures are my forte. I have always been much at home with figures, calculations, creative mathematics."

"What did you invent?"

Ernesto thought for a second. A strange light widened the pupils of his eyes, moving me to wonder what would come next; the sharp beam of intelligence alive and clear, or the glossy stare of alienating obsessions. To my growing interest and relief, it was

73

the former which lit up his next remarks. "I have found a way of getting all of the wild life to reproduce itself," he declared with quiet pride. "It is a radically new system. A splendid invention!"

"All of the wild life?"

"Yes. And here is how it works. First, you take one specimen from each group: a lion, a giraffe, an elephant, a hippopotamus, any animal you can find in the jungle. Then, you put them all together in one great pit in the ground—according to my calculations, this pit must be at least one thousand metres long, five hundred wide, one hundred and fifty deep—you put them all together in this pit, as I said. Finally, you slam the lid on, very tight." He paused.

"Then what happens?"

"They procreate."

"All of them?"

"That is correct. What actually takes place is this: when all these animals have been in this pit for some time, and the lid has been kept on tight, they all end up believing there is no other world outside this pit they are in, and as they realise this, they begin to feel the need to create another world, so they procreate. Quite simple, is it not?"

"Yes," I echoed. "Quite simple indeed."

Ernesto looked worried all of a sudden. "Excuse me, Roberto," he said, reaching in his pockets for a pad and a pencil. "I think I made a slight error. Let me see. . . ." He sat at the table and began feverishly writing down a lot of figures.

I walked away as discreetly as I could.

CHAPTER FOUR

If a manicomio was the pit Ernesto had in mind,
then his theory was sound in one respect at least: you
make friends quickly in an asylum. And I realized this
the moment Don Pedro cheerfully waved for me at the
other end of the long corridor. Frantic as I was to see
Valerie and to get out of here, I felt I must take time to
say good-bye to some of the inmates I had met during
these few hours.

The first one I ran into was my conspirator friend
with the raincoat buttoned up to the chin. He was most
distressed that I should be leaving so soon after we had
made contact, he said, now he and I would never
accomplish our mission. I told him I would do my best
to keep in touch from the outside, so perhaps we might
accomplish our mission some other day.

"Understood," he said. Then in a whisper he added,
"I shall always bear in mind that you call yourself
Robert Goulet."

"Chesterfield?" I ventured.

He gave me a knowing look. "Filter-tip."

I nodded that I got the message. He winked,
looking very pleased with himself.

As I left him, I noticed that my neighbour Jaime
was standing by the door to the dining room, waiting

75

for me. But he did not look at all happy. "You promised, Roberto," he whined reproachfully.

I hastened to tell him how sorry I was that we could not be together on the four o'clock train to Soller this afternoon.

He shook his head sadly. "But we had made a deal."

"Listen, Jaime," I said, "as true as your own sister put you in here, I will come back in a few days and bring you some of your own oranges from the valley."

Jaime went on shaking his head sadly. His old eyes were moist when we said Adios.

Then turning around at the call of my name, a few steps further, I saw Ernesto hurrying to catch up with me. He, too, appeared genuinely sad to see me go. It wasn't everyday that a writer came to the Manicomio, he said mournfully. Afraid he might have made a mistake in the measurements for his pit, he asked if I would consider staying a little longer to give him time to verify the figures, as I must have the correct dimensions before I wrote about his theory.

"I appreciate that very much," I said, but he needn't worry as the exact size of the pit interested me less than the whole idea of his invention. Besides, I promised, I would check with him again before deciding to mention it in my next book.

That seemed to cheer him up a little. We shook hands. Then I continued up the corridor.

About half-way to the door of Don Guillermo's office, where Don Pedro stood patiently waiting for me, I passed a group of men huddled together against the wall. "Good-bye, senor. Good luck, extranjero," they cheered. I returned the good wishes and shook hands with every one of them.

Feeling rather good, I had a look in the garden to

see if my other friend was there, the one who went around beating up guardias after one drink too many. But I could not find him. So I continued on my way. Then as I walked past the door to the infirmary, I saw him standing in line with several inmates, some of whom held their pants down while others rolled up their sleeves. I waved good-bye. In response he broke into a fit of shadow boxing, as if a guardia had suddenly appeared before him. "Like this, honourable friend," he shouted. "A left and a right! Give them a good one for me, first a left, then a right, like this. Watch!" Two brown-frocked men grabbed him by the arms. He started screaming. They were giving him a shot, when I looked away and hurried on.

Don Pedro now greeted me with a slap on the back. "Come," he said. "Your senora is waiting."

"Thanks for everything you've done for me," I told him.

"What! Are you leaving?"

"Of course."

"Who said so?"

"You just said my wife is here, didn't you?"

"Ah, Roberto!" he scolded. "Be reasonable, my friend. Give us a bit more time. You have only been here twelve hours."

We entered Don Guillermo's office. I knew I was going to say something nasty the moment we faced each other again. But Don Guillermo was not here. A secretary was transcribing something from a tape recorder hidden in the top drawer of the desk.

"How do I sound?" I asked her, as I recognized my own voice.

She did not look up from the typewriter.

"What's the matter?" I pressed on. "Don't you like the sound of my Spanish?"

"Patience, Roberto," Don Pedro snapped. "Do not become nervous." He opened the other door and nodded me to go in. "See you later."

I now found myself in another small office. Then suddenly all I could see was Valerie. Something tender and familiar inside me quickened to an urge to embrace her, but at the same time a sense of distance, separation, held me back. She seemed to be leaning forward, almost on tiptoes, waiting for me to make the first move. Love was all over her face, but touched with a deep sadness.

"I'm sorry," I heard myself mumble.

We fell in each other's arms for a long moment, not saying a word, eyes shut. When I looked into Valerie's face again, the sadness was still there, but she was smiling bravely now.

"Let's get out of here," I said.

"I just talked with the director, and he says we must first get a final report from the guardias before you can be released. But don't worry. He promised to let you go today."

That's a likely story, I thought to myself: Don Juan is playing for time, looking for a way to keep me here as a guinea pig for Don Guillermo. But I did not want to tell Valerie about that; she was upset enough already. I pulled two chairs and we sat down.

There was so much to tell. Not knowing where to begin, we interrupted each other in overlapping bursts of cross talk the main points of which took some of the pressure off our minds at least. The children were all right, she had just left them with Robert and Beryl Graves in Deya. No, my face didn't hurt, it looked worse than it felt, really. Yes, it had been a hell of a night in Fornalutx, but no matter, Rafael was fine, only a broken nose, and nobody else was hurt. Of course the whole village was up in the air. But again no matter, we would take a vacation off the island and everything would be forgotten when we came back to Balitx. And how did I feel? What about this place?

"But it is *you* I am worried about," I insisted. I could see that Valerie had been crying a great deal. One side of her chin was swollen and she had put a thick coat of make-up over the bruise. I had a sickening sense of being a first-rate bastard. "Tell me what happened, please."

"Let's not talk about that for now," she said.

"Please, darling, it's terribly important that you tell me everything. I can't go into all the reasons why, it's too complicated. But if you really want to help—listen, after Santa Marta, what did happen?"

Valerie gave out a long sigh. Then after a moment to collect her thoughts, she began. "It was past seven o'clock and you were not coming back. So I walked down to the plaza thinking you might have driven off to Soller or to the Puerto. But the car was still there. I looked in at the Centro, then at the Deportivo. Finally I tried Santa Marta and Pierre told me you had been drinking with Katie but had left shortly after the last bull on television, about fifteen minutes before. I walked back to Balitx and waited until about eight.

"Then as it was getting dark, and you still didn't show up, I decided to go and see Katie. She was in the middle of preparing dinner, but luckily nobody else was there. She told me you had only two drinks with her at Santa Marta and sounded all right when she left you, though a bit upset about your work, she said. She was very helpful; seeing how worried I was she dropped everything and got Benito to drive her to the Puerto, where Theo had gone for a short swim before dinner.

79

Together they went out looking for you all over the Puerto and even in Soller.

"In the meantime there was nothing I could do but go back to Balitx and wait. And I worried, of course, knowing what mood you were in when you left. By now I was pretty sure you had walked down to Soller and gone on drinking till you didn't know what you were saying. I was sure you had gotten into some sort of wild argument with Mallorquines—well, you know how you can carry on, and how nasty they can be with foreigners!"

"Yes," I thought aloud, remembering my painter friend Donald Crowe and how five or six of the locals had beaten him up one night when he was so drunk he could hardly stand up. His wife had found him at the foot of a lemon tree the next morning and it had taken him one week in a hospital to recover.

"Dinner was ready," Valerie was saying. "I had made a spanish omelette and laid the table on the terrace as it was lovely and warm, and I was still waiting, when all of a sudden I heard someone calling out from the entrada. I rushed down. It was Pierre, trying to carry you up the steps. So I gave him a hand. But you could not stand up. You could not speak. You were white as a sheet. Oh, God, you weighed a ton, my poor darling! We tried to carry you all the way upstairs and put you to bed, but you wanted to lie on the floor in front of the fireplace. Pierre had been on his way to the stables to feed Pamela when he found you face-down in the ditch a short way up the road from the cafe, and it was only because you moaned that he found you, he said, it was so dark. He couldn't understand what had happened; all the way up to the house you kept telling him you were not well. Of course he thought perhaps it was his fault. He said he had noticed you did not look

80

well these days and were inclined to argue a bit much after a few drinks, and he supposed it was because you were working too hard on your book. So he was very sorry to have given you those last two drinks, but he had not wanted to upset you, he told me, you kept insisting you were all right. You even left the cafe walking quite straight, he said.

"Anyway, I put a blanket over you, as you were lying on the sheepskin in front of the fireplace and it was getting chilly. Then I was sitting there waiting, hoping you might come to and let me take you upstairs to bed before Katie and Theo came in and found you in such a state, when suddenly you woke up, just like that, and jumped to your feet. There was a fierce, terrible look in your eyes and you started shouting, 'Where is Rafael? I'm going to kill him!' I tried to talk to you, calm you down, but you couldn't hear me. It was as if you couldn't even see me, you didn't know who I was, or where you were. I took your hand to lead you upstairs, but you shoved me so hard I fell back in the chair. Then you started down the stairs shouting that you must kill Rafael, rid the village of that monster, and all sorts of things. You were really gone, my darling. I have never seen you in such a state. I ran after you across the entrada, caught up with you at the door and tried to hold you back. Then the next thing I knew I was lying on the stones outside senora Mayol's house, my chin was sore, and you were not there any more.

"I ran for help. Luckily enough, Theo and Katie were coming up the steps on their way to Balitx just then. They already knew what had happened at the Centro, but wouldn't tell me everything. They merely said you had an argument with Rafael and the Guardia had stepped in and both of you were now at the

81

Cuartel. They wanted to come with me to the house and we would all wait for you.

"By this time the whole village was out. Everybody was there, even the little children, looking sleepy and lost and wondering what this was all about. Inside the Centro and the Deportivo the men were drinking and arguing. They had even turned off the television as nobody was watching any more. And on the plaza it was like both a fiesta and a funeral at the same time. The women had gathered in small groups all over the place and they were whispering and shaking their heads, pointing fingers at me now and again. When I started down the steps, they all fell silent and turned, then just stared at me as if they had never seen me before. And as I went on down I could see the cruelty and the hatred on their faces. Oh, it was horrible! They were so silent I could almost hear my own breathing. I don't think I've ever been so frightened in all my life, facing that mob all alone down there.

"Then Theo rushed over to join me, and together we walked on to the Cuartel. People shouted at us to go back home, stay there and lock the doors. You had gone mad, they screamed, and they meant to protect their women and children, things of that sort. There wasn't a single person who came forward to offer help. Oh, now I really know what they can be like.

"Well," Valerie went on after a pause. "When we finally arrived at the Cuartel, the guardias told us you had just been taken to the jail. I could not understand. The Cabo, Pepe and Jesus, even the other guardias, had always been so friendly with us, I just couldn't believe they would turn against you all of a sudden and do a thing like that. Surely they could see you had been drinking, I told them: why didn't they simply take you home and we would have put you to bed? Then Theo tried to explain how bad it was to leave you in that jail in the condition you were in. But they wouldn't hear a thing. The Cabo said you were not drunk. You had gone mad because you were overworked, he insisted. We argued with him. I told him Pierre himself had carried you home from Santa Marta. We pleaded with him. But he just wouldn't give in. As far as he was concerned you were mad and you had struck someone and that was that. And he meant to do his duty, which was to protect the people of the village, he said. He even told us we should thank him for putting you in the jail, as the village people would lynch you if you were still out on the plaza right now. Finally, after at least two hours of arguing and pleading, he gave in a little and said Theo could go down and look in on you; the village doctor was out in Palma, he said, and legally he could not refuse a doctor's visit. Well, it turned out that it might have been better after all if Theo hadn't gone there to see you."

"I know," I said. "I can remember swinging for him. I think I missed, though. But why I should have wanted to strike Theo, I just don't know."

"The point is, on coming out of there Theo simply told the Cabo you were not well. Now, you know Theo's Spanish is not very good. The Cabo took his comment to mean that he, the Cabo, was right, you had gone quite mad. And the next thing we heard the ambulance had been called and you were being taken to Palma. It was Pierre himself who came in to tell us, about midnight.

"So we all rushed down to the Cuartel hoping they would tell us the name of the hospital. But what do you think? They almost threw us out, told us to go home and stay there and lock the doors as the people in the village were still pretty angry. And I never found out where you were until about eight o'clock this morning,

when I ran into the Cabo's wife at the tienda. She
looked embarrassed, rather sad about the whole thing. I
asked if her husband was up as I wanted to know
where they had taken you in Palma. Then I think she
wanted to make up for what he had done. She more or
less said I shouldn't bother with him this morning, then
told me you were here."

I said: "So you really think the Cabo turned
against me?"

"I am quite sure," Valerie said. "Though I haven't
the slightest idea why he should want to hurt you."

Wondering aloud what it could be, I recalled how
Pepe and Jesus and the Cabo himself had behaved in
the ambulance. Then we both agreed that something
was very wrong indeed: this was much more serious
than I had thought at first.

Valerie said, "When I passed in front of the Cuartel
this morning I saw several men with the Cabo and it
looked as if they were signing some sort of paper.
Rafael was there, too."

"That must be the denuncia," I said. "The charge."

"But don't worry about it," Valerie hastened to add.
"I have explained everything to Robert Graves and he
says I am to tell you to stay calm and wait. Alfredo,
Robert's lawyer, will take care of it so you will be out of
here before tonight. Now—"

The door opened. It was Sor Catalina. She wasn't
smiling any more.

"Senora," she said. "If you will follow me, please,
the director would like to talk with you at this
moment."

"Go ahead," I said to Valerie. "I'll wait here."

"I love you," Valerie said with a brave smile, then
was gone.

All alone in the small room, now, going from one

84

bare, whitewashed wall to another bare, whitewashed wall, as I paced up and down across the window bars shadowed on the tiled floor, I thought about the whole messy situation and tried to see how it might have been avoided, how the fire might have been put out before it was too late. But after a while there was nothing I could see but the face of Rafael—he was smiling in that treacheous way of his that was a grin, a sneer.

"Agreed, senor Roberto," he was saying. "Only, now you must pay me double; once for myself, and once for Antonia."

*   *   *

The background of Rafael's appearance in my life must be set four years back, soon after my arrival in Mallorca. At that time my first wife and I had decided on a trial separation, so she had remained in Connecticut with my teen-aged son and I had come here with the first draft of a new novel that needed to be almost completely rewritten. As I had not arranged for a place to stay, Robert Graves invited me to Deya, where I spent a few weeks while looking for a house in the Soller Valley. During that time a friend of Robert's unexpectedly decided to return to England with her children. She had a small house in Fornalutx. I went to see it, liked the village at first sight, took a lease for one year. The house had modern plumbing, was completely furnished, with linen, dishes and all, and there was a room upstairs where I could work. There were three cats, but they had to go back to the mountains soon after I moved in, as I did not like cats. There was also a maid, but whether I liked the idea or not she came with the house and that was that.

Her name was Antonia. She was a good-looking little woman in the mid-thirties, vivacious, full of adventures, an excellent cook, delicate with flowers and

85

plants, very good at mending my socks but not so good about leaving dirt in dark corners behind the furniture. She had the now dreamy and now wide-eyed look of a woman who likes men and will go for a quick tumble if you hurry up to close the windows and lock the front door. I saw it at once, but kept my distance—not so much from a lack of interest, however, as from a built-in sense that certain things in life do not mix well.

And so Antonia, by staying out of my bed, remained a good maid, and we got along fine. After a long day of work she would bring a pot of camomile to my study and sit there telling me what had happened down the mule steps today, the latest gossips, who among the foreigners had just returned, or left, even what Don Cristobal had preached in his sermon this Sunday. She would sometimes talk about herself, too, so that little by little I finally got to know about her thirteen fiances, including her latest one, Rafael, with whom she had broken off only a few months before I arrived in the village. "He is uncouth, not delicate, not fino," she said. "And so jealous! My God, he would never permit me to work for you if he were still my fiance. A terrible man!"

He certainly did look terrible, I thought the very first time I saw him, wondering what a delicate and "fina" little woman like Antonia could find in him at one time. He was the one you would pick as the perfect bastard or the ugly man of the plaza. Tall and powerfully built, he walked somewhat like a sailor in a storm at sea: the top of his head was a bare strip of glossy skin between tufts of negroid hair, he had a mean mouth, a large nose, enormous ears, and he could see with one eye only. He was so ugly indeed that I might have felt sorry for him if he had not already declared war against me, publicly swearing to drive me

86

out of the village before the year was over. I was
sleeping with Antonia, he asserted at the Centro, and
one of these days he was going to prove it.

At first I did not pay much attention to what I
heard, even though much of it came from Antonia
herself. Nearly every week she would show me a new
letter he had just sent her about what he intended to do
to me in order to save her honour. As he put it at the
end of each letter, she was still his fiancee in his heart
and so he must save the reputation of the children they
would have together after she had become her sweet
loving self again—"pronto" he hoped.

Rafael's jealous rantings soon echoed out of
Fornalutx and to the four corners of the valley. And the
foreign colony had me tagged as the lecher of the
village, what have you. Still I refused to pay attention
to all the noise, telling myself that people would soon
get bored with the subject and drop it. But Rafael did
not intend to stop there, obviously. He now took it into
his head to wait for me in the dark of a porch, or
behind walls, when I returned home after a few drinks
at Santa Marta. Pierre himself had spotted him a few
times and told me about it, adding that perhaps I ought
to be careful as Rafael had a history of violence in the
village.

And the situation remained the same until I left for
America almost one year after I had first set foot in
Fornalutx. I bought Balitx just before leaving,
intending to return the following year and live in it. By
that time Antonia would probably have gone back to
Rafael, they might even get married, I thought, and
although I did not like the idea of losing her as a maid
I still preferred this to the prospect of being haunted by
Rafael through the mule steps of Fornalutx when I
came back.

Balitx is a twenty-four room posada dating back a few centuries and traditionally regarded as the manor-house of Fornalutx. It stands next door to where I had spent that first year with Antonia as my maid, and my immediate neighbour to the right is Rafael himself. Balitx had not been lived in for twenty-five years when I bought it, yet I was able to move in the day I came back from America, one year later.

Balitx needed a lot of work, of course, but for the time being I intended to limit myself to what was strictly necessary. Electricity and plumbing must be installed as soon as possible. Not that I expected a family to join me soon, my fifteen-year old marriage having just ended in divorce; but I was anxious to take as little time as possible away from writing.

Antonia meanwhile had gone to London to work for her former employer. She was due to return with the family next door sometime in the spring, I was told. I was told also that Rafael was up to his old tricks again, claiming that Antonia had left Fornalutx because of a broken heart and swearing again at the Centro that this time he was going to bury me in cement long before the toilet was installed in Balitx. There seemed to be only one solution to this whole problem, then. And I acted upon it immediately it crossed my mind. One night I arranged to meet Rafael on the terrace of Santa Marta; after a few drinks we struck a deal and shook hands on it—he and his men would do the work on Balitx.

For a while all went well. The work Rafael and his men did was good, the bills were honest and paid promptly and in all appearances Rafael and I were good friends. Often at the end of the day I would have a drink with him at the Centro, and it was heart-warming to feel that the whole village looked favourably upon this change in our relationship. I was welcomed in several of the local homes, there were many in the village who dropped the senor when they addressed me, I organised free English classes in Balitx, and generally speaking the doors of my house were open to anyone who cared to come in for a drink or a chat, a love letter to be read or written, a tool to borrow. Several members of the foreign colony warned me now and again that it wouldn't do to mix so much with the locals. Someday I would end up at the losing end of it, they said.

And they turned out to be right, although it took me a long time to realise it, just as it took me a long time also to realise that the pact I had made with Rafael was not viable. True, I had never felt that I could trust him fully, somehow. This was partly due to his look; it was physically impossible for him to meet you straight in the eye, you could not tell which one of his eyes was dead and which one was alive, so in the end you never really knew what was on his mind. But there was something else. Each time we happened to be alone after a few drinks he would somehow shift the talk over to Antonia, mainly to assert again and again that it was he, not she, who had broken off their engagement. Then to justify his position he would tell me about her having had an illegitimate child at eighteen and an abortion at twenty, things I had already learned from Antonia herself and I did not want to hear all over again each time I was with Rafael. I also noticed that I would increasingly ask myself, particularly on waking up in the morning, whether or not I had told him last night that I had gone to bed with Antonia while she worked for me. I sensed that he would feel a lot better if I confessed to it. He wouldn't stop baiting me until I gave him some sort

89

of satisfaction, I thought. And at times I was tempted to do so, if only for the sake of making him drop the subject once and for all.

Meanwhile it dawned on me that the work on Balitx was slowing down in almost direct proportion to my growing reluctance to discuss Antonia with Rafael. If for instance I had cut him short in the middle of it, last night, then his men were likely to start work at eight-thirty instead of eight, this morning. Or he would take two men off the job for the afternoon. Even worse, he would declare that we had suddenly run out of cement in the village and so drop all work for one day or two. After several months of this it began to look as if Rafael's masons would never leave Balitx. Yet I was still holding out against what I had now begun to regard as a power of evil I was determined to defeat in the end.

Then came Valerie, and we got married. I stopped going to the cafes in the evening. I also put an end to the English classes. The work on Balitx slowed down to a snail's pace. There was no choice but to give Rafael an ultimatum. In reaction he kept away from work for a whole week, drinking at the Centro all day long. I finally had to fire him and get a mason from Soller to finish the work.

Weeks later, the new mason was still repairing the mistakes Rafael had made with the septic tank, the dining-room chimney and the floor of the bathroom, when Rafael sent me his own closing bill. He was charging almost twice the number of hours spent on the job, the wages had gone up, so had the cost of cement; it was altogether a very dishonest bill. So I refused to pay it and told him to get a lawyer and we would fight it out in court. His reply was an invitation to meet on the mule steps and he would break my face, and so on and so forth, followed by a series of threats entoned to the four corners of the valley. Clearly, it was time I did something about it.

And I tried. Several times I invited him to drinks, which he accepted. Then I would say to him, "All right, Rafael; I'll pay your bill in full. But let's have peace. How about it?"

"Agreed, senor Roberto," he would say. "Only, now you must pay me double: once for myself, and once for Antonia." And he would just sit there smiling in that treacherous way of his that was a grin, a sneer, until I got up and walked away in helpless rage, raging to hit him.

*   *   *

"Hey there! Stop hitting that wall," someone was shouting behind me. "You are going to hurt yourself."

But I finally had Rafael's face where I wanted it, and I knew my blows were landing now and I must finish him off so he would never again sneer at me.

"Roberto!"

Then all of a sudden Rafael was gone. And Don Pedro was standing at the door.

"Dios Mio!" he sighed out. "You *are* a violent one."

I did not know what to say. My hands were sore.

"What's the matter?" he pressed on.

"It's . . . it's that fellow I hit last night," I tried to explain.

"Don't you think you have hit him enough already?"

"I'm sorry," I said. "Please don't tell Don Guillermo about this."

"Come, amigo," he said gently, firmly stepping up to me.

"No." In a flash I knew that he was now going to take me back in there as one of them. "I must stay here

91

and wait for my wife," I said.

"The senora has just left. She will come back this afternoon."

"That's not true," I began to protest.

But at that moment Sor Catalina came in. She cast a quick, chilly glance at me, then whispered something to Don Pedro, who frowned and now looked me up and down as if he had never seen me before.

"Come along," he said abruptly. Sor Catalina opened the door and nodded that I should do as I was told.

I obeyed, thinking: "So this is it! The director must have heard from the Cabo of Fornalutx. Or maybe they rushed down the denuncia by special messenger." We crossed Don Guillermo's office. "What is it?" I heard myself ask.

Don Pedro said nothing. Sor Catalina pretended I was not there any more. They both seemed to be in a hurry.

"What's going on?" I asked once again.

Don Pedro's reply was that haunting, familiar sound of his great keys as he locked the door behind me. I saw the long whitewashed tunnel of the corridor stretching before us. Sor Catalina hurried on ahead. Don Pedro soon caught up with her. The two of them began whispering animatedly as they went on, turning back to look at me now and again.

Convinced that they were discussing my case, I decided to follow them in the hope of catching at least a few words. There was nobody else in the corridor. You could hear distant sounds of talk and dishes from the dining-room at the other end. I saw Don Pedro insistently pointing at his watch. Sor Catalina seemed to be telling him not to hurry so. I was beginning to wonder what all this might have to do with me, when suddenly they turned right and disappeared into the infirmary.

I hurried on, till a short distance from the door. I slowed down to silence my footsteps a little. Then I heard Don Pedro plead softly aloud, "Now, please, now." On tiptoes, almost, I took a few more steps up to the door. "Yes, yes," Sor Catalina was saying. I thought I could hear Don Pedro breathing heavily, almost panting. There came a faint whisper of rustling skirts. Then slowly, silently, the door was shut.

I hesitated a moment, looking up and down the corridor. There was nobody around. I simply could not resist. Hot in the face, and feeling my heartbeats quicken with a strange excitement, I bent down to get a peep into the room. And here, framed in the Moorish arch of the keyhole stood Don Pedro with his pants down. He was leaning forward a little, when a rush of black skirts suddenly shuttered him off, then just as I thought the skirts were beginning to move again so that I might finally see what this was all about, I felt a hand on my shoulder.

"Better get away from here," someone whispered down my back.

Anticipating a blow from a brown-frocked man the moment I straightened up and turned, I just waited, holding my breath and feeling trapped, utterly miserable, ashamed of myself.

"Hurry up."

I turned.

It was a very old man, and he looked worried on my account. His fly was open; he had been coming out of the lavatory when he caught me. In a confused state of relief and lingering shame I followed him quietly away from the door. When we were at a safe distance up the corridor, I thanked him.

He said, "If you get caught spying on those two, they'll put the earphones on you."

"What's that?"

The old man stuck his forefingers to his temples and did an imitation of trigger-pulling with his thumbs. Every wrinkle in his face suddenly twisted and twitched in an expression of intense pain. Then he assumed a bland, stupid air, and, shaking his head, said: "Now you don't know nothing. You ain't seen nothing. The picture's gone, see. Burnt out."

I thought of my guardia-hating friend and what he had said about electro-shock treatments. It didn't seem possible that Don Pedro and Sor Catalina should do a thing like that to a patient who happened to have caught them in the act. Nor, for that matter, did it seem possible that Don Pedro should be in there now pulling down his pants for Sor Catalina. Anymore than it seemed possible that I should be peeping at them through the keyhole. Or that I myself should be here in the first place, come to think of it.

"Christ!" I thought out loud. "Things are getting muddled up!"

"What was that you said, son?"

"I said this is a spooky place."

"What do you expect? This is a manicomio. We're all nuts, aren't we?" He winked knowingly. "Now look at that one, up there." He nodded ahead of us.

I saw my conspirator friend, head lowered in deep thought and walking in our direction while keeping very close to the wall. I hoped that he would not see me.

"Comes from Sineu, a tiny village in the center of the island," the old man said. "Nice, clean-cut lad he was, they tell me, working in the fields with his folks and keeping his nose clean and just about to get married to a nice cousin of his. But then one day he comes to Palma, a Sunday afternoon it was, and he sees a movie about a secret agent during the war. That was in nineteen forty-six. He's been here ever since." The old man paused, then nodding sadly, added, "Well, he should never have left the farm, is what I say."

My conspirator friend had just spotted me. He made a quick turn. "Robert Goulet?" he said, and waved at the old man to leave us alone.

"What do you want?" I asked him, saying to myself: now don't get impatient, bear in mind this poor fellow is crazy and you're not, remember what Don Pedro said about going along with them, don't get mad, stay calm, let him come closer if he wants to, play the game, it will make him feel better.

"What's on your mind?" he said.

"Nothing," I said. "What's new with you?"

"I waited for your message."

"Chesterfield?"

"Yes. Filter-tip?"

"They didn't have any."

"No message?"

"No."

"Did you make contact?"

"No."

"Been out?"

"No. There's been a mistake. But I will be leaving this afternoon."

A shade of suspicion darkened his look. For the first time in our strange relationship he seemed to feel ill at ease.

"But don't worry," I added. "I'll have our message back to you by tomorrow night the latest."

Suddenly he looked his old self again. "Chesterfield?"

"Yes. Filter-tip."

"And don't forget you are Robert Goulet."

"I will not."

"Because if you do, I won't."

"Fine."

"For the sake of our mission, we must always remember that you are Robert Goulet."

"Fine, fine."

"Robert Goulet, see."

"Fine, fine, fine," I burst out in exasperation. "But stop reminding me, for Christ's sake, you're driving me nuts." Then angry at myself for blowing up, I marched off.

He ran after me. "Robert Goulet!"

I dashed into the dining-room, where I promptly lost him as I picked my way among the tables to where I found one with an empty chair. Everybody stared at me. It was easy to imagine what they must be thinking. Had it not been for a reviving shot of self-control, I might well have burst out again, proclaiming in high tones of righteous vindication that there was nothing wrong with my head, I was still here because of some mistake with the documents upstairs, the director himself had promised to release me this afternoon, so let nobody stare at me as if I had really gone nuts! The three inmates at the table I had picked looked up from their plates of white rice. One of them pulled the empty chair out for me. They all smiled that I was welcome.

"No," I shook my head. Then telling myself that I wasn't hungry anyway, I walked off in a hurry.

At the door, I came face to face with my neighbour Jaime.

"Roberto!" He spread out his arms.

My first reaction was to shove him off and keep going, but he seemed so thrilled to find me here again

that I quickly mellowed down to sighing out, "Yes
Jaime. Now what is it?"

"So our little deal is still on?"

"Sure," I told him.

"What happened?"

"A bit of a mix-up in the documents. But it's all
being straightened out right now."

"So we will leave together on the four o'clock train
this afternoon?"

"It's a deal."

"Oh, I am glad you came back, Roberto! I knew you
would not let me down."

"Fine," I said. "But let me pass, now. I must go
somewhere."

"Of course. I suppose you have a great deal to do to
get ready. I will be waiting. Hasta luego, Roberto."

"So long, Jaime."

The corridor was filling up with inmates pacing up
and down for digestion while waiting for the brown-
frocked men to unlock the doors to the garden. The
playroom at the other end looked empty, so I decided to
head in that direction. Falling in line with the men, I
kept my head down, my hands behind my back, in the
hope that nobody would notice me and I might be left
alone. There were faint pleading requests for a
cigarette now and again, but I pretended to hear
nothing. And when my conspirator friend brushed past
me, muttering my name once more, I simply nodded
that I got the message and went on my way. There was
a lot on my mind. But to sort things out I must first
pretend that I was not here, somehow. This place had
already begun to have such an effect on me that I could
no longer think clearly without making a conscious
effort to do so.

"Now let's start at the beginning," I told myself,

trying to remember what on earth I might have done to the Cabo to make him turn against me all of a sudden. But I had barely heard the whispering echo of my own thoughts when, looking up at the sound of keys nearby, I saw the door of the infirmary open, then Don Pedro coming out, followed by Sor Catalina. The sight of them at this moment only added to the confusion in my mind.

Don Pedro had removed his white frock and put on a sports jacket. He no longer appeared to be in a great hurry. Nor did Sor Catalina: she in fact seemed more calm and rather pleased with herself. After what I had seen through the keyhole, at this point there was only one conclusion that made sense, and in a flash I remembered a host of dirty jokes of the type we used to tell about the nuns and the priests in Quebec. But the next second, when Don Pedro looked at me as he passed by, that conclusion was reversed in my mind and I now faced something even more difficult to believe. He was looking at me straight in the eye, but there was not the slightest sign of recognition in his look, there was in fact nothing but a glossy stare and I had the impression he could not even see me. It was the same look I had seen in the eyes of Ernesto, my neighbour Jaime and my conspirator friend.

I was still standing there watching Don Pedro walk away towards Don Guillermo's office, wondering if there was something wrong with him, or with me, instead—which one of us was going mad, was I beginning to see things, now? when Sor Catalina asked me, "Have you had something to eat, senor Roberto?" with a sweet smile on her lips.

"Yes," I said.

"Perhaps you would like to walk in the garden?"

"I could use a bit of fresh air."

"Are you not well?"

"I am all right."

"Then do cheer up," she said kindly. "The senora will come again this afternoon. You will probably be talking with your lawyer also. So do make an effort and cheer up a little, won't you."

"Thank you," I said. "I'll be all right. Adios." And I hurried away from her, suspecting that she was trying to find out if I knew what she had been up to with Don Pedro inside the infirmary.

I walked up the corridor towards where the great doors had just been unlocked. The inmates were beginning to pour out into the garden. I would find a cool spot in the shade along one of these high walls, then just lie down in the grass, I decided. I wanted to be alone. I needed to think things out. Yet I knew that I must not think too much. I wished that I could find someone to talk to. But there was nobody.

"Everybody here is nuts," I thought to myself. "Just plain nuts." Then as I heard myself hammering away at the word "nuts," it dawned on me that this word no longer sounded the same now as it had before I entered this place. I tried the others: crazy, mad, loony, off your rocker, and around the bend; then madhouse, loony-bin, and nuthouse. But it was the same for all of them. This was nothing to laugh at any more. These weren't the sort of words to be used in a light vein. Even the Goulet's amused tolerance in referring to the family as "Not well" now had an ominous quality about it. And suddenly I was afraid, the way you get frightened when you can no longer laugh at the silly things that used to scare you at one time but that you had learned to laugh at as a defence mechanism. It was like believing in ghosts suddenly at forty.

So I was glad to see the daylight, as I stepped past the doors. The sun had never seemed so bright. I could

99

feel the good heat of it rapidly warming my back. In a moment I heard someone calling for me. I turned quickly.

It was my guardia-beating friend. But I could hardly recognize him. He lay in a heap against the foot of the wall, one shoulder raised as if to protect his face from a blow, his hands dangling in front of his chin, and his watery eyes stared at me with fear and pleading. I stepped up to him, wondering what they had done to the poor fellow.

"Please go away," he moaned. "You come here, bring back the bad dreams, and now look—they give me a shot—they burn my muscles away and I am left with the bad dreams and I cannot hit back. It is your fault, honourable gentlemen."

It was hard to know what to say. I could sense that his mind was clear and that he was suffering a terrible anguish. I thought of offering him a cigarette, but did not have any left. I wanted to do something, anything to help him a little.

"Please go away," he went on moaning. Yet there was no hatred nor resentment in his eyes, only pain, helpless suffering.

So I stayed next to him, thinking this was perhaps what he needed, if not what he actually wanted, at bottom. His pleading subsided after a while. Whining softly aloud, he seemed to be trying to get off to sleep across resurging images that made his face twitch and sent spasms down his legs. I did not leave him until he had become silent, still.

I then took the path in the shade along the building and headed towards the bright sun beyond the maze of gravel walks. There were a few inmates strolling silently in head-bent solitude. Hundreds of others were sprawled all over the place in the hot light.

I desperately wanted to go to sleep, too, forget that I was here. Coming out of the bright sunlight, I picked a spot in the shade of a tall carob that grew on the other side of the wall. Then I lay down in the grass and tried to imagine that I was back in Balitx.

We were finishing lunch in the lazy shade of the vine on the terrace, with Valerie against the greengage in bloom. It was the end of the Albinoni tape on the music system and we were feeling drowsy in the hot siesta sun, quietly happy now as we had not had a row. And it felt good to be waiting for who would give the first sign to go upstairs; where it was cool in the green shade of the tall shutters and we knew the children were asleep in the nursery, so that we could be together now, lucky—something moved, or made a sound.

It was Ernesto, "May I be with you?" he said.

I nodded yes.

"Sor Catalina sent me to cheer you up," he said. "You must proceed cautiously, Roberto. Do not permit yourself to become depressed."

"I was not here just now, and I did not feel depressed."

"That is the spirit, Roberto. Your mind should be somewhere else. You must live only in your imagination while you remain here. There is no other way. Remember what I told you about my theory: when you are in the pit, and the lid is on tight."

"You should have been a writer, Ernesto."

"Que va, Roberto!" He sat up against the wall. A look of childlike musing came to his old face. "I like figures, you see, creative mathematics. I am not good with words."

"Nevermind," I said. "Do you know anything funny?"

"You want to hear stories?"

101

"I get frightened when there is nothing left to laugh at."

"I used to know a great many jokes at one time, but it always seems there is nobody to tell them to, so I forget them all, being here so long, I suppose."

"Then tell me about Don Pedro," I said.

"What do you wish to know?"

"Everything."

"And you promise you will tell nobody about it?"

"Yes."

Ernesto lowered his voice to a whisper. "He is a very sick man, actually. They say he takes morphine. But I hear it is something even stronger. He gets a shot every day, just before going home at two. And the strange thing about it is, he does not need the drug while he is here, he seems to need the drug only in order to face the outside world."

"I see."

"Another thing," Ernesto went on. "It has to be Sor Catalina who gives it to him, nobody else. And what is even more strange, he will take the shot only with his trousers down in front of her."

"Very odd."

"And do you know where she gives it to him?"

"No."

"In the arm."

"Queer fellow, isn't he!"

"Naturally, Roberto. You and I are the only sane people in this whole place."

"Are you sleepy?"

"Are you?"

"Yes."

"But please do not fall asleep just now. In case you do leave this afternoon, there is something I must tell

102

you before you go. Listen, Roberto. Are you listening?"

"What is it?"

"About the length of the pit. I have verified my calculations again and it is not one thousand metres, that would be a little too long, we must make it no more than seven hundred and . . . ."

Now it felt good in the cool shade of the shutters, upstairs in Balitx.

CHAPTER FIVE

I could hear someone calling me across barren fields littered with boulders and rocks, where I was running for my life under a blinding sun, pursued by clamouring hordes of Fornalutx people with bleeding noses, twisted mouths, fierce, bloodshot eyes and tight fists beating the air in wrath. Wanting to duck under the stones they were throwing, I stumbled, but picked myself up at once and, frantic for air, went on running in crying despair of ever reaching the safety of that olive grove up the steep mountainside, where the voice kept calling, "Here, extranjero, up here!" Then just as I thought one of their flying stones was about to land on the back of my head, I woke up with a start, in a sweat.

It was cool in the silent shade of the high wall now and the shadows of carob leaves were on my feet. Ernesto had left. The fog of sleep lifted, then I could see the shade spreading to the maze of gravel paths in the center of the garden. Most of the inmates had gone indoors. From the open windows of the playroom came faint waves of gaudy sounds—the television set was on.

Then realising how late it was, and wondering why Valerie had not come yet, I sensed that something had gone wrong. But I did not want to think about that. And then maybe it wasn't so late after all, I told myself; there was still a patch of sunlight at the other end of the garden. A man was standing there with his back to the setting sun, making an impassioned speech to his own shadow creeping up the wall. A cloud of stupor soon blurred the edges of my waking. More fatigued than depressed now I leaned back under the carob tree and once again tried to return to Balitx in my mind, carefully avoiding all thought of Fornalutx people for fear of drifting into another nightmare of violence.

But again that voice called out in the distance, "Extranjero." And someone else shouted, "Roberto."

I jumped to my feet, now fully awake. A brown-frocked attendant and a fat little man were coming towards me across the sun-and-shade line. I started up to meet them. The attendant turned and walked back to the playroom, leaving my visitor alone. After a few more steps I recognised Alfredo.

I had met Alfredo several times in Deya, the last occasion being Robert Graves' birthday party in July. He was about thirty-five, charming in a boyish way and very popular with the foreign colony along the Deya coast, where he had a summer chalet and sailed a small boat on weekends. He had been handling Robert's affairs in recent years and Robert himself had told me he was a good lawyer. I had heard also that many foreign residents of the Soller Valley used him when closing a deal on a house or when in need of a permit to keep the car in Spain for another six months. The son of a prominent member of the Falange, Alfredo had contacts, people said he could fix anything—*En Espana todo se arregla* is a popular saying in this country, and Alfredo was the man to prove it. For my part, I had never thought of him in terms of what he, a lawyer, might do for me. Naturally, it had never occurred to me that my troubles with Rafael might land me in the

105

asylum; which is why the sight of Alfredo now only added another touch of the incredible to the nightmare of finding myself in this place. His face was aglow with that same boyish, wide-eyed gladness with which he would greet you at a party. The only thing missing was a glass of Fundador in his plump little hands.

"Que tal, Roberto?"

"Very well, Alfredo. How goes it with thee?"

"Stupendous!"

It was kind of him to pretend that we were not here. He gave no sign of noticing the cuts and bruises on my face. So I went along with him. "And how goes it with the boat?" I asked.

"Stupendous!" he exclaimed with pride. "I entered the regatta in the Bay of Palma last Saturday, and finished second."

I congratulated him, then said, "When are we going out sailing together, the two of us?"

"Tomorrow, if thou wishes, Roberto. They will release thee tomorrow before midday."

"Is that true, friend of mine?"

"With a bit of luck, it shall be so."

"Let's walk," I said.

Then he told me all about it, as we took the center path that ran the length of the garden to where the inmate of a moment ago was still addressing his own shadow on the wall. It had been a full day for Alfredo. After getting our version of the story from Robert in Deya, he had gone to Fornalutx and talked with some of the people who were at the Centro when it happened. He had also dropped in on the Guardia Civil and seen the Cabo himself, who refused to brief him on the details and seemed determined to make the most of the incident. The complaint was signed and a guardia on motorcycle had already taken it to the judge in Soller.

The judge was a distant cousin of Alfredo's father, so it would have been possible to stop everything right there and then, but the old judge had already acted on the complaint and the papers were on their way to the Manicomio by the time Alfredo reached Soller. The only thing to do then was to pull strings in Palma.

"Which is what I have been doing all afternoon," Alfredo said, eyebrows raised to indicate this was one problem that was not so easy to fix.

"I wonder why," I thought aloud.

"The law is very strict on this one point," Alfredo explained. "Once you are committed to a mental hospital for judicial reasons, you simply must remain committed for at least two weeks, which seems to be the time they need to find out if you really belong here."

"Hell!" I said. "It's plenty of time to make a man turn loony, once they set to work on you."

"Then perhaps that explains why we have such a law in the first place," Alfredo whispered, suddenly secretive and looking back over his shoulder as though we were being followed. "After all, judicial reasons are not always very different from political reasons, are they?"

"But Alfredo!" I exclaimed. "They told me thy family was of the Falange!"

"Que va!" He put one arm around my shoulders. "Mallorca has always managed to end up on the side of the winner, Roberto. This time it is the tourists we are interested in. Now, political troubles are not good for tourism, so we keep away from political extremes." He winked. "Understand me?"

"I get it."

"Anyhow, the law, as I said, is so strict the director himself can do nothing about it, even if he thought you were perfectly well and could be released immediately. So, the only way to get you out of here is to petition a High Court judge to find you not guilty. And this cannot be done until a specialist in forensic medicine has examined you and certified that you are sane— which I am sure he will do without hesitation in thy case, Roberto."

"Thank you, friend of mine."

"I have already seen one, as well as talked to the High Court judge who will hear our case," Alfredo went on. "Now this judge was a good friend of my father's, he is a partner in a chain of hotels on the island, he himself had a drinking problem at one time, so we can count on him to be understanding towards a poor tourist who lost his head after one drink too many. Only, he may want to ask you a few questions about your statements regarding the testicles of our Head of State. According to the Guardia Civil, you are supposed to have said most unflattering things about the guardias and their connection with Franco's private parts. Now what will you say to the judge?"

"I don't know," I said. "I can't remember exactly."

"Splendid!" said Alfredo. "That is precisely what you must tell the judge. You do not deny, you do not admit, you simply cannot remember. Clear?"

"Clear."

"As for our special doctor, well, as we say in Spain, *todo se arregla*, provided, provided—"

"How much does he want?" I asked rather bluntly.

"Three thousand," Alfredo whispered. Then he hastened to explain what a great favour this specialist was doing us by accepting to certify me a sane person on a Saturday morning, these few precious hours when he usually went fishing off the coast of Cala D'Or. It was an open secret of course that the eminent doctor also had a young woman, Danish, who had a chalet in that part of the island, and so—"

"And so it is all fixed?" I said.

"For three thousand, yes," Alfredo said, then promptly added, "God willing, friend of mine."

It all sounded so easy that I wondered if Alfredo was feeding me a tall tale to cheer me up. I could almost hear Don Pedro giving him a few tips on how to deal with the kind of people who ended up in this place. And this made me think that perhaps Alfredo had talked with Don Guillermo, who might well have briefed him along the same lines.

We left the garden. Alfredo went on about our special doctor's double life, finding the whole thing rather spicy, yet anxious to point out that such goings-on will sometimes put quite a strain on a family man's pocketbook, and so we must be understanding, must we not? I agreed with him, adding that there was nothing particularly shocking about it so long as our case could be fixed. But at the same time I was finding it increasingly difficult to hide the suspicion that was growing in me as we entered the building and headed for the small room where I had seen Valerie in the morning. Alfredo simply sounded too confident, a bit too jovial, even; I could not shake off a pack of apprehensions, haunting doubts, awkward questions about the real purpose of his visit. I was in fact more worried than ever by the time we shook hands and he left with a reminder not to worry, I would certainly be out of here by noon tomorrow.

"By the way," I called him back. "Any message from Robert?"

"Well yes," he suddenly remembered. "He asked me to tell you to keep calm. He and Beryl are coming to see you on Sunday. They'll bring along some of the

109

friends from Deya, a whole group, in fact. So cheer up, Roberto. Adios."

"Thank you, Alfredo," I said. "Adios."

Then immediately he had left it occurred to me that he had made a mistake. How could he say that Robert was coming on Sunday, when he knew, or at least had assured me, that I would be released tomorrow, Saturday? Surely he's got his days mixed up, I thought.

Next I came face to face with Sor Catalina at the door. She was carrying a suitcase, my own green one. "Su esposa," she began.

"But where is the senora?" I interrupted.

"Now do not become excited, senor Roberto," she said firmly. "The senora brought this suitcase and tried very hard to see you just now, while you were with your lawyer, but the director gave strict orders that you are not to receive any more visitors today. We have already made quite a special in your case, you know. So be a good patient and come along, now. We are moving you to another ward."

I picked up my suitcase—it seemed rather heavy—and followed Sor Catalina up the long corridor. We did not meet a single inmate on the way; they were all watching television in the recreation hall. And this cheered me up somewhat; or, rather, I was relieved not to have to face any one of them at this stage. We soon came to an enormous dark-wood door which Sor Catalina unlocked with a key twice the size of the crucifix she wore on her chest. It opened onto another corridor, but more cheerful than the one we left behind. There were doors on both sides and what looked like a bright and spacious lounge at the far end. From somewhere half-way up on the left a nun appeared and came towards us. I was being officially admitted into Ernesto's special ward.

"But why bother to change wards for one night only?" I thought, then promptly gave up trying to understand.

My room was a small, whitewashed cell that contained a cot, a washbasin, no mirror, a closet, a straight chair and a table, then a tiny, high-set window with iron bars that let in a green touch of twilight. I dropped my suitcase onto the cot. The two nuns immediately zipped it open for a thorough search of what Valerie had sent me. There were oranges, enough to last a couple of weeks at the rate I usually ate them, more chocolate bars than I could digest in six months, enough sets of underwear and pairs of socks to last me a winter trip to Quebec, one full ream of paper, a handful of number-two pencils, a toothbrush, one large tube of toothpaste, plus what I slowly counted as thirteen books altogether. One nun took the pencils and the other the toothbrush, explaining that I could use the toothbrush any time I wished provided I asked for it and then brushed my teeth in the main washroom where an attendant was on duty around the clock. As for the pencils, well, we would have to wait until Don Guillermo gave his approval. Speaking in Mallorquine, Sor Catalina then said to her campanion that although I seemed a bit worried over the length of my stay in the Clinica Mental de Jesus, I was, in every other respect, a very good patient. "But a bit thin," remarked the other, speaking directly to me in Castellano. They called her Sor Petra, she said, and went on to promise that I would look a lot fatter by the time she was through with me. Then before leaving, Sor Catalina expressed the wish that the Good Lord might remain with me, and Sor Petra announced that she would return in a

111

short while with a "bisteck"—the senora had insisted that this was my favourite food and I must be given at least two a day, regardless of the cost.

"Do not think, darling. Try not to worry. And keep busy. See you tomorrow. *Keep busy.* Love, Valerie."

The note was at the bottom of the suitcase. I read it several times, trying to understand it in connection with all the things Valerie had sent me.

"Why send all this stuff if she really believes I am going to be released tomorrow?" I wondered. The books in particular bothered me; not only were there enough for a month or two of steady reading, but as I looked at the titles, one by one, it dawned on me that I had read every single one of them, a fact that Valerie could not possibly be unaware of.

Then suddenly I knew it, the way you know you are going to choke when it all blocks up in the throat and you start up for a bit of air. This was it: I was here for keeps, both Valerie and Alfredo knew it and they were trying to throw dust in my eyes!

All I could see, when I looked up beyond the iron bars, was a small patch of darkening sky faintly brushed with red. It was the same sky as over the Soller Valley when the sun hits the rocky flanks of the Puig just before sinking into the sea behind the Puerto. I grabbed the chair, climbed onto it, and, holding the bars so tightly that I could feel the cold iron slowly warming up in my hands, I tried, tried very hard to imagine it was tomorrow, now, and I was leaving.

*   *   *

Leaving a place you cannot recall having entered is disquieting. It seems unreal, vibrant with bewildering suggestions of people and events unrelated, lending the moment a nightmare quality of total alienation. And in my case this mood was deepened a thousandfold by the

112

layout of the asylum itself, for if ever the concept of alienation was given reality in the choice of a location for a mental hospital, this was it.

The Clinica Mental de Jesus was in Palma, yet not in Palma. The high walls surrounding the institution would stretch nowhere groping for links with lower stonewalls or pavements of the city; instead they ended next to a small forest, a thick limbo of green vegetation studded with great outlandish pines. Trees make for excellent soundproofing along highways on approaches to cities and towns. That is how thorough the architects had been in isolating the asylum from the city— nowhere must the agonizing screams from one place meet with the lively sounds from the other, this being conceived as a perfect no man's land of silence. It reminded me of Ernesto and his invention for the mass procreation of all the specimens in wild life: if this patch of green silence was the lid to be slammed tight over the pit he had in mind, then I had a pretty good idea where his theory might have come from.

I was sitting in the front of the car, with Valerie behind the wheel and Alfredo on the back seat. We had not exchanged a word since starting down the narrow road that ran straight between plane trees for a few hundred yards and then became a maze of winding curves presumably designed to prevent any look back at the place once you had left it. I wondered if Valerie and Alfredo were keeping silent because of being as impressed with the setting as I was.

Nowhere in Mallorca had I seen a spot of land so green. This was not the dull green of olive groves, nor the deep, dirty green of orange and lemon trees, nor the brownish green of the carob, nor the pale, sickly green of the Mediterranean pines. This was the cool, clear green of the Irish countryside touched with a fresh glow of springtime grass under a bright midday sun. And the red earth was flooded with pools of sunshine scattered among irrigation ditches full of water flowing fast and surfaced with silver wrinkles that shot a million darts of light up among the pines. It was theatrical, unreal, fairylike.

The sight of these pines sent me back to my native Timberland in Quebec. Then tasting the sharp resin in each breath of air, I was climbing down the wooded banks of the Saint-Maurice towards where my brother and I had left our canoe the night before.

All of a sudden I saw one brown-frocked man appear on the right, then another one near the road, and then two more a little further on, and after a while I counted the vague shapes of at least half a dozen inmates bent over irrigation ditches in postures of children sailing miniature boats over artificial lakes in city parks. Not one among the inmates looked up at the red Mini as we drove past, but every one of the brown-frocked men did, then nodded at me. It seemed strange to see them and not hear the sound of their keys. I wondered if Ernesto was among the inmates. I looked for him left and right, as we drove on, wondering at the same time why I should be looking for him now.

Now they were all gone, quite suddenly, it seemed, as we rounded another sharp curve in the road. This one turned out to be the last, for we came out of this no man's land, next, very abruptly. Then we saw Palma, white and Moorish and hot and gaudy and loud in the haze of noon.

*   *   *

A knock at the door made me turn away from Palma in the sun. Suddenly I was back in the dim twilight of my cell. Sor Petra walked in with a tray. I

114

climbed down from the chair, saw the "bisteck" Valerie had ordered.

"You necessitate this," Sor Petra said firmly. "Now you eat it."

I did not like that nun. Her looks bothered me; she had dark, bushy eyebrows, a wart on the chin, with one long hair growing straight out of it, an adolescent's moustache that drooped at the ends, giving her mouth a mean twist. She was not half as gentle as Sor Catalina. She was in fact much too bossy, I thought. And I promptly decided she was a lesbian, that I would get along with her no better than with the Quebec nuns who had brought me up through regular beatings every month or so from the ages of six to fourteen. I said rather harshly, "What about the utensils?"

She shook her head.

"A fork and a knife," I insisted.

"Forbidden."

"You mean, I am supposed to eat with my fingers?"

"Yes, then wash your hands very well afterwards. Cleanliness has much importance in our treatment. It cheers one up to feel clean."

I said, "I am not hungry."

"Good appetite," Sor Petra said curtly. Then after a quickly mumbled "God be with you," she was gone.

So petty a detail should not have bothered me so, perhaps, but in the state I was in I simply could not cope with it. A great weight settled upon my shoulders, as of something too heavy to bear, and in a moment I could feel it spread to my arms and then all the way down my legs, sending throughout my whole body a sensation of extreme fatigue. I had a creeping premonition that I was entering the last stage of a desperate struggle from which I was bound to come out utterly defeated, and with it came that sour,

115

overwhelming helplessness of deep humiliation. I wondered why I should feel so humiliated over such a small thing—there is no shame in eating with your fingers, I told myself—but that only intensified my helpless, bitter resentment.

So I just sat there for a long session of morbid ruminations, staring down at the piece of meat in the paper plate, lost in a stupor as all my thoughts centered upon one inescapable conclusion. "Eat away at a man's pride," I repeated to myself. "And that's bound to break him down. A bit of humiliation now and again, that is how they make you turn, slowly, bit by bit . . ."

It was pitch dark in my cell, and my fingertips told me I had nearly filled the ashtray with butts, when I finally stood up and decided to look around the ward in an effort to change the train of my thoughts. I put on a pair of slippers, took a fresh pack of cigarettes and walked out shutting the door without a sound.

The corridor seemed endless and ever narrowing in the dim light from overhead bulbs burning so low you could almost count their filaments. The floor was patched with odd triangles of pale light where cell doors were left ajar. The air smelled of dirty socks, ammonia, stale urine and something like camphor.

As I went on towards the lounge, I grew aware of a strange silence that sounded like a deep moaning sigh rising from underground. Or did it come from beyond the walls filtering down from the wards upstairs? I fell to wondering if this was an hallucination, when Sor Petra came out of the infirmary with a syringe held needle-up in one hand and a wad of cotton-wool in the other. She did not see me. I stopped dead against the wall and waited till she had disappeared into a room three or four doors up ahead.

Then I continued towards where I could see the

116

corridor ending in a frame of flickering, silver-blue light. In a little while I detected the voice of the television newscaster. The evening bulletin was on. I entered the lounge keeping my back very close to the wall, afraid to intrude.

About a dozen inmates sat in various stages of absorption in what the screen showed them. I recognized Ernesto's white head among the ones immediately in front of the set; he had a pad on his lap and now and again his head would lower a little as he jotted down something. One man near him kept his back turned to the set and was running a tumultous commentary on the news, presumably, but to himself alone. I could hear someone snoring hoarsely in the middle of the room. After a while I detected a light tapping noise as of a stick hitting the floor at regular intervals, then as my eyes grew accustomed to the blueish dusk of the place I spotted an old man walking slowly along the opposite wall and picking at the floor with a cane that obviously had a metal tip at the end. Farther on, I saw a very tall man dressed in a white smock and standing absolutely still in the back of the room, his arms folded, his chin up, his gaze wandering loftily over his charges. "So this is part of the extras you get in this special ward," I thought; the attendants wore white.

In a moment the ceiling lights came on and the set was turned off, as the news ended and Bonanza was about to begin. I took a cigarette and struck a match, but did not have time to light it before a pair of fingers out of nowhere daintily picked the matchbox from my hands, and a high-pitched voice lisped over my shoulder, "Sorry, senor."

It was the white-smocked attendant. And I was tempted to protest: Ernesto had told me they were

117

allowed matches in this ward and Sor Petra had not removed them from my cell. But the man's countenance and looks were such that I remained speechless at the sight of him at close range. He was built like a football player, but stood like a mannequin modelling a tight skirt—the right foot slightly forward, toes pointing out, a faint suggestion of swing in the left hip, a lofty, withdrawn look in his pale blue eyes and a smile of self-satisfaction touched with disdain. Decidedly, I thought, this was just about the worst specimen I had ever met of what some people call "a mad queen." And he seemed to be most anxious that I become aware of it as quickly as possible. He now struck a match and offered to light my cigarette, saying in a half-sweet, half-officious manner, "Nothing personal between us, sweetheart. Rules are rules, you know. You will find there is a reason for everything in this place, after you have been here for some time. Meanwhile I shall ask Don Guillermo if we can make a special in your case." He pinched my ear gently. "Thou art so sweet," he added. "Now smoke. Do have a puff."

I might have struck him, if I had had a drink or two. Or perhaps I would have kidded him along. I do not know. Suddenly I blew out the match he was holding up to my cigarette, then walked away without a word, while he stood there glaring at me, his lips contracted in a prissy, cruel look.

"Got a light?" I asked Ernesto, whom I had just spotted coming towards me from behind this strange white-smocked attendant.

"Ola!" Ernesto gave me a warm, Spanish-style embrace, nearly crushing the cigarette down from my lips. "Que tal, Roberto?" he exclaimed. "It makes it such a long, long time since I last saw you. And how I think about my writer-friend all the time! And about

118

the measurements for our pit! Remember? Even now, a moment ago, I was still revising my figures."

"Enchanted to see you again, Ernesto," I lied. "Now would you please give me a light?"

He quickly pulled out his Zippo. "So they brought you back?"

"I never left."

He gave me a blank look.

"But tomorrow is the day," I went on. "So I will have been here just about one full day altogether."

Ernesto shook his head violently, as if to put things back in order up there. Then suddenly he said, "God of mine, now I remember! Of course, Roberto, of course. That was last year, in the other ward. Last year it was, I remember now."

"Ernesto," I tried to refresh his memory. But in vain.

"I am so glad they moved you here with us at last," he went on. "Splendid, Roberto, splendid."

"I cannot say I am going to like it in here," I said. "Even for one day, the other ward seems better. Sor Catalina is all right, so is Don Pedro. Now take this attendant here. I don't like the looks of him."

"El Maricon?"

"The maddest queer I've ever seen."

"But do not let him upset you," Ernesto said. "He is really gentle when he wants to be, and there are some among us for whom he will do a special favour once in a while, if you understand what I mean. Do not worry yourself, however; he will not bother you if he feels you are not one of his kind. Only, you must never cross him. He is terribly strong, could easily take on the whole of us with one arm only. A real bull of a man, for a maricon."

119

"Fine," I said. "I'll try to keep out of his way for tonight."

"That is the spirit, Roberto. You must remain a good patient so we can spend some time together, the two of us. Oh, how enchanted I am to see you again! Now we shall be able to talk, and talk. Perhaps I will help you with your writing, then you can help me with my inventions, and we will—"

"Ernesto," I cut him short. "Who is that man staring at us?" I nodded towards the old man with the cane, who was now standing only a few feet from us, his eyes fixed upon my mouth in an expression I could not understand: there was pleading in his look, a touch of anguish, a fleeting dart of menace. "What does he want from me?"

"Your cigarette," whispered Ernesto.

I immediately took the pack out of my pocket to offer him one.

Ernesto held back my hand. "No," he said. "That would only upset him greatly. It is your cigarette butt he wants." He gently led me away towards the corridor, going on confidentially. "That is the famous Louis Coll, you know, one of the greatest contrabandista on the island at one time, and perhaps one of the richest men in Mallorca today. We call him El Cenicero."

"You mean, the ashtray?"

"That is correct. They put him here years ago when the government decided to take over all contraband activities on the island and he refused to go along with the police because they demanded too much of a cut. He was not easy at the beginning, I remember. Most violent he was, till they gave him the right medicine to calm him down—several sessions with the earphones, I hear—so now he is a nice, gentle old fellow, quite harmless, as you can see." The stick came tapping along behind us. "All day long he goes around the ward picking up our cigarette butts," Ernesto continued. "They say he even gave Don Juan a large sum to make sure there would never be an ashtray in this ward as long as he lives here. Then every night, before going to sleep, he straightens out and unrolls all the butts he has picked up during the day, keeps the paper in one pile and the tobacco in another, until he has accumulated a considerable stock for those days when the picking is poor. He then rolls the butts back together, very neatly, and goes around the ward dropping them here and there, so he always has some butts to pick up with his stick." Ernesto paused, then added, "Not so crazy after all. It is merely a question of inventing your own system, as I once told you. How do they call that, outside, when they refer to us? Something like, there is method in his madness?"

"Yes," I said. "I heard it said before." I dropped my cigarette butt on the floor, which brought a sudden increase in the speed of the tapping sounds behind us, until there came a pause, then I knew the "ashtray" was satisfied.

We had walked down the corridor almost to the door of my cell. I did not want to invite Ernesto in for a late chat. Besides, I had just become aware of a strong need to pay a call to the lavatory. So I used this as an excuse to say good-night to him right there and then. "Where is the vater?" I said.

"Is it for pipi, or kaka?"

"Just tell me where it is."

"Over there, the third door on the right," he said, growing impatient. "But listen, Roberto; it depends on your needs. You may have to ask the attendant."

"To hell with him," I said. "Good night, Ernesto." And I hurried away.

121

Now, there are delicate situations in life that call for patience or humour, or both, if one is to avoid unpleasant consequences. But patience, let alone humour, were the last virtues I could resort to at the end of this day. I was too exhausted emotionally, as well as physically. And that may well explain why my needs of a moment ago had become so imperative by the time I reached the men's room. In any case, had I been a little patient with Ernesto, I might have found out what he meant by asking the attendant first—there was no paper.

"Paper!" I shouted at the top of my lungs.

In a moment the white-smocked "queen" came rushing over. He took his modelling stance in front of me, then with a faint snort of disdain, said, "So my sweetheart is having an evacuation?"

"Yes," I said. "And I would appreciate having it in private. Just get me some paper."

"Sweet Mary mother of us all!" he chanted, raising an eyebrow. "Why did you not ask me, first?"

"Just get me the roll, and leave me alone."

The angrier I grew, the more he seemed to enjoy it. "Senor," he said calmly, "Did it ever occur to you what terrible things people can do with a roll of toilet paper?"

"You know what *you* can do with it."

"Good God of mine!" he exclaimed, and his hands went to his backside in a lewd gesture.

Now I might have laughed. And I wish that I had thought the whole thing funny. But it was the indignity of my predicament which got the better of me. I was up on my feet, next, quite forgetting that my pants were down. Then ready to strike him, I shouted at the top of my voice, "Paper, I said, paper, do you hear, paper, paper—"

"Very well," he cut me short in a calm voice. "Very well, senor; only, you must indicate how much you necessitate."

I sat down again, feeling despair and helplessness and bitter humiliation driving me to the point of tears. "Please," I said. "Stop torturing me. Just bring me a bit of paper to wipe my ass. That's all I ask of you."

"I understand, senor," he said. "But again I must insist that you tell me how much you necessitate. I cannot give you the entire roll, you see. That is against the rules."

"Just bring me what you want."

"Would half a metre be sufficient?"

"How do I know?"

"One full metre?"

"Anything you want," I said, exhausted. I could feel the rage moving in on the wake of the fatigue and helplessness. I was sure I would not be able to endure much more of this. "Hurry up. Bring me one metre, then."

"Some ass my darling must have!" he said with a snort. And at the same time he turned to go, giving me a lewd, quick shake of his backside.

And that is when it happened. In one motion I pulled my pants half-way up, high enough for a good swing, and gave him the hardest kick I had ever driven up anybody's behind. He let out a little cry, and turned. I caught a terrible light in his blue eyes. He did something to me that I did not feel. I do not remember what took place next.

I recall lying down on the cot in my cell. I was on my stomach and my pants were down. Something cool touched one of my buttocks. Sor Petra was bending over me. I felt the needle go in.

"This will do you some good," she said firmly.

"Yes," I agreed weakly. "This will do me some good."

"In this place," the high-pitched voice lisped, "there is a reason for everything."

"Yes," I agreed with the white-smocked attendant. "There is a reason for everything."

"Including you being here, senor Roberto."

On that thought, no longer worth fighting against, I felt, I drifted to sleep.

CHAPTER SIX

"Violence, violence, and more violence," Don Guillermo declared, nodding gravely over a fresh report added to my file on his desk. "The pattern is set most clearly. And perhaps forever, unless. . ." He looked me straight in the eyes. "Roberto," he added, dropping the formal Don or Senor and speaking in a gentle tone of compassion, "You are in the center of a circle. That circle is narrowing. You are caught, absolutely trapped." He paused, kept his eyes fixed on my face in an expression of hope that I might agree with him.

I was still half asleep; either from the shot Sor Petra had given me, or due to the blow from the white-smocked attendant, or as a result of both, I could not tell. They had just pulled me out of my cot and Ernesto himself had helped me to get dressed, I was so drowsy and my back felt so stiff I could hardly bend down or lift my arms. "Well now," Ernesto had scolded me; when a man had enough intelligence to write books, he should also have sufficient brains not to pick a fight with a bully the size of our white-smocked *Maricon,* especially in the *Vater* and with my pants down; so I had received a rabbit punch and I would know better the next time I needed an evacuation—"Promise?" Then Don Pedro had come to fetch me, wearing a look of uneasy concern over my conduct, and I had walked

125

down the long corridor seeing nobody and hearing nothing but the voice of my conspirator friend who kept reminding me that I was called Robert Goulet; which did not bother me so much this morning as it had yesterday, somehow, leaving me less harrassed than amazed, until his voice dissolved into Don Guillermo's in a vague, haunting sequence as on the blurred edges of an inexplicable dream. For the moment I was grateful to be allowed to sit down and rub the back of my neck, trying hard to wake up fully while nodding wearily over anything the psychiatrist might say.

"I am enchanted that you agree," he went on. "That is our starting point. It is most important that you understand this. You need help, Roberto. That is why you are here. And I can help you, but only if you see clearly into your illness and are willing to co-operate with us. Understand?"

"What time is it?" I said.

Don Guillermo sat up, and the look of compassion dropped from his face. He set his elbows firmly on the edge of his desk. "Senor Roberto," he snapped, "The time of day should be the least of your worries, believe me. This morning especially." And in the same breath he launched into an upbraiding recall of my recalcitrant behaviour at yesterday's interview.

"To hell with you!" I thought. Besides, I detested him so much that the very sight of him was helping to clear my head. In a little while I could tell just about what time it was. The skin on his face was tight and dry, his cheeks glowed faintly seared as from a fresh rubbing with after-shave lotion, while every gesticulation he made as he spoke agitatedly with his hands sent a whiff of cheap cologne towards me. So he had just come in, I decided, and I must be his first patient; which made it between ten and ten thirty. To

126

hell with him, I thought: in another hour and a half or
so I would be out of here for good.

"Then you were caught in a fierce act of pugilism
against the wall next door," he was saying. "I hold Don
Pedro's report right here. Would you like to see it for
yourself? No? Well, I understand. None of this comes as
a surprise to you, that is why. Nor are you unaware of
what the incident means, all that it reveals about your
secret obsessions. You even begged Don Pedro not to
tell anybody about it; which proves that you are fully
aware of your condition. You know perfectly well what
is wrong with you, what haunts you, what drives you to
violence; that is to say, when it matters very much that
you should know, then you do know, do you not?"

I thought of an obscenity to throw at his face, but
held back. "Keep calm," I told myself. "Don't say a
word. Don't even look at him. Just let him go on. And
think about noon, in another hour from now."

"And last night," he went on, "what happened in
the *Vater* last night?"

I said nothing.

"You were not drinking. So you know what came to
pass. You remember perfectly well, do you not?"

I remained silent, picking at my nails in an effort
to keep calm.

Don Guillermo waited a while. Then as I still
refused to speak, he let out a long sigh, sat way back in
his chair (his high heels must now hang about the floor,
I thought) and crossing his hands like a priest in deep
meditation he began a fresh recapitulation of what had
happened in Fornalutx.

"That bastard!" I thought. "He's really enjoying his
job in this place."

And why not? It was quite a combination, come to
think of it. Now a friend, now a policeman, now a

127

how American publishers handle an author's title when promoting his novel.

"Why not see things as they are, Roberto?" he said kindly. "There is no shame in being ill. Nor is your condition a particularly rare one. Obsession with violence is a disease of our times, especially in America. You are a fairly representative product of your own time and environment. And by the way, perhaps that explains the success of your first novel." He paused, as if this last statement were a question.

"What time is it?" I said.

"Your very refusal to see it is pathological. It constitutes the proof of your illness. It also proves that you are aware of your condition."

"Could you not tell me what time it is, at least?"

"And now," he announced sternly, and stood up; "we are going to make a final verification. A new experiment, we might call it. It comes directly from America, your own country, Don Roberto; so you need not be afraid. We have come a long way from the Inquisition." He smiled.

"You son-of-a-bitch," I thought, but said nothing.

He pressed the button on the wall behind his desk, then pulled a measuring tape out of the middle drawer, speaking to an unseen audience somewhere above my head. "In this test we refer ourselves to the Circles of Protection," he explained. "In other words, we measure the patient's tolerance to physical intrusion, and this gives us an idea of his violence potential. You will see for yourself in a minute."

Now I was afraid. I knew it by the sudden quickening of my heartbeats, although I could not tell exactly what it was that frightened me. Also, for the first time this morning I began to doubt that Valerie and Alfredo would come and fetch me before noon.

There were all those books Valerie had sent me, then Alfredo's apparent mistake about Robert's visit on Sunday. I fell to wondering all over again if both of them had given me a tall tale in order to cheer me up.

"Would you please stand up," Don Guillermo said.

I did, then looked back over my shoulder to see if Don Pedro was coming in answer to the buzzer.

"And stand right here," Don Guillermo went on, pointing to a spot on the floor halfway between his desk and the door.

Obediently, and telling myself to keep calm, I did as I was told, feeling somewhat ridiculous and knowing with increasing disquiet that this must be a trap he was setting up for me.

"Now do not move."

I stood still, taking deep breaths in an effort to relax. I needed desperately to smoke, but could not bring myself to ask Don Guillermo for a cigarette, I hated so much the very sight of him. In a moment the door behind him opened. For a flash I hoped it might be Valerie, or a nun coming in to say that my senora was waiting for me in the next room.

It was Don Juan, the director. He hardly looked my way, let alone greet me. In a quick manoeuvre that seemed pre-arranged between the two of them the measuring tape passed from Don Guillermo to Don Juan.

"What time is it?" I asked Don Juan.

"Proceed," he said to Don Guillermo.

The latter turned to me and said, "I am going to approach you now." He was standing eight to ten feet away from me, with Don Juan next to him.

"What time is it?" I asked again.

"And you will tell me to stop when you feel I am coming too close," Don Guillermo went on, moving

131

slowly towards me, while Don Juan kept his gaze fixed on mine in a wide-eyed, avid look of search.

My eyes fell on the men's shoes, and the sight of their high heels made me smile.

"Here?" Don Guillermo asked, after a second step in my direction. Then taking a third one, "Here?" he asked again.

I went on smiling, but consciously so, now, rather in an attempt to disguise the way I felt. At bottom I could tell that I was getting nervous in almost direct proportion as the space between Don Guillermo and myself went on decreasing—now quite rapidly, with the next step he took.

"Here?"

"Go ahead," I said, surprised at the note of defiance in my voice.

He moved forward another pace. "Here then?"

"No."

"Do you mean I should stop here?"

"Go ahead," I nearly shouted, my heart thumping.

There was nothing but friendliness in the way Don Guillermo was advancing towards me, and his voice was growing gentle with each step nearer. Yet my knees were beginning to tremble and my mouth was quite dry by the time he had reduced the space between us by another foot or so.

"Here?"

"Go ahead," I shouted against my will. My hands were clenching into fists.

Don Guillermo took another step, very slowly, then said, "Here?" And he continued his advance before I could reply.

"At your own risk," I then heard myself shouting at the top of my voice, and backed off a step or two.

Don Guillermo stopped. Don Juan hurried to

measure the distance between him and the spot where I had stood a second before. Don Guillermo then took my pulse. And before I knew it the two of them were back behind the desk, inviting me to sit down again; the experiment was over, Don Guillermo declared.

"And it is most conclusive," Don Juan said. "Your Circle of Protection has a radius of a metre and a half, nearly sixty centimetres more than that of the most violent patients we have here, and almost double that of the average non-violent person on the outside. Therefore your intolerence to physical intrusion is much too high for me to sign your release. Our first diagnosis is confirmed. Good day, senor Goulet. Your wife will be permitted to visit you twice a week. See you later, Guillermo."

When the director had gone, I said to Don Guillermo, "What time is it now?"

He sat down, looked at his watch, lit a cigarette, said nothing.

"You will not break me down this way," I heard myself mutter angrily.

The smile of scorn appeared on his lips once again. And that is when I became convinced that he must hate me even more than I hated him. "Better keep calm," I said to myself. "Say anything he wants. Agree with him. Play for time."

"May I have a cigarette?" I said.

"Now that is better," he said with a friendly smile, and offered me a filter-tip. "There is something else I desire to tell you. But we will not make any progress unless you co-operate fully."

"Go ahead," I said.

He thought a moment, then said, "Do you wish to be cured?"

I nodded yes.

"What are you disposed to do in order to be cured?"

"Anything."

"I mean, to be rid of the obsessive images that drive you to violence?"

"Anything you say."

"Well," he rubbed his chin, "here is the treatment we contemplate for you, Roberto. But do not be afraid. Trust in me. You are an intelligent man, I have much respect for you, so I shall explain . . ."

*   *   *

Electroshock is a treatment employing electricity to produce convulsions similar to . . .

"The earphones!" I thought about Ernesto and how he had warned me that they would put the earphones on me if I stepped out of line.

Little is known about the actual dynamics of electroshock therapy, so we are really working in the dark on that score, although unquestionably success has been observed in cases of involutional melancholia and other depressive conditions. . . .

"The earphones!" I thought about the old man who had caught me spying on Don Pedro and Sor Catalina in the infirmary yesterday afternoon. They would slap the earphones on me if ever I told anybody about what I had just witnessed through the keyhole. "Then you ain't ever seen nothing. You won't ever know nothing."

The therapeutic possibilities of electric current passing through the brain were discovered accidentally by two Italian doctors, Carletti and Berni, who, while treating epileptics, noticed that with some of their patients who happened to suffer from schizophrenia also, there often was a marked improvement in the schizophrenic condition after an attack of epilepsy. In other words, the state of shock induced by the epileptic seizure appeared to erase or destroy whatever images were responsible for the schizophrenic behaviour. So . . .

"Look out for those earphones!" I thought about my guardia-hating friend with the countenance of a prize-fighter and the scraggy, burnt out limbs from being locked up in half a dozen manicomios throughout Spain. "There are dreams they cannot take away from you, honourable friend. There are dreams that just won't burn."

In order to produce convulsions similar to those of epileptics, it was found that a small charge of electricity. . . .

"Marie!" I thought about my cousin and how they had made it possible for her to live without her six illegitimate children. Eight months in the Quebec asylum, then so many shock treatments, and she had come out a new woman. She never again mentioned any of her children, whom the priest had placed in separate orphanages through the province. She never again threatened her father with the kitchen knife. She now went to mass every morning, looked after her father and mother very well. A new woman she was, my cousin Marie. And as I thought about her now, I knew those shock treatments had done a lot more than just kill the mother in her.

Seventy to one hundred and fifty volts, for a length of zero point one to zero point five seconds, should prove sufficient for a final application. The patient is made to lie on a firm, straight surface, with a pillow placed lengthwise across the litter and against his buttocks. This is to prevent any injury to the spine during the convulsions. A mouth gag is also needed; as a rule we use an applicator thickly padded at one end with gauze, which we place in such a position that the canine teeth bite on it as the mouth closes during the seizure. The mouth opens widely when the convulsions begin, so we

135

apply upward pressure on the jaw to prevent dislocation and keep the gag in position to prevent biting of the tongue or lips when the jaws close. Also, during the convulsion, we hold the patient to prevent dislocation of his arms and legs, and . . .

"Poor Timothy!" I thought about our friend Spencer and how he looked the day I visited him at Saint-George's in London just after he had gone through that therapy. I asked him if he wanted anything the next time I would come to see him. Yes, he said, he wouldn't mind The Observer. So I had gone back the next day, Sunday at noon, carrying the paper and a box of chocolates. But he had just jumped out the window. They allowed me to have a quick look at him in his room on the third floor: he looked the same as he had the day before.

A convulsion may last for about one and a half minutes. But six attendants are needed. Two assistants stand on opposite sides and apply pressure on the patient's shoulders, each with his other hand grasping the wrist of the patient's arm nearest him. The arms then are flexed and held firmly but not immovably against his chest during the convulsion. Another assistant applies downward pressure on the pelvis. Two more hold the patient's legs, with one hand above, and the other below, the knee. An experienced person must stay with the patient until full consciousness returns. Finally, as a rule in this place, shock treatments are given only in the morning before breakfast.

*   *   *

"Have you taken your breakfast, Roberto?"

"No," I snapped, jumping to my feet. "And I'm not going to take your treatment either. There is nothing wrong with me. The guardias put me in here by mistake, and you've done nothing but try to break me

136

down. I'm still all right. You can't treat me as if I were insane. You can't—"

"Sit down," Don Guillermo said calmly.

"My wife and my lawyer are on their way to fetch me now and a judge in Palma has accepted to hear my case this morning. Let me out of here so I can pack my things."

"I said sit down, senor Roberto."

I started for the door leading to the ward, but it opened suddenly before I could put my hand on the knob, and Don Pedro appeared.

"Roberto!" he exclaimed with a great show of joyful surprise, the way you greet an old friend you haven't seen for years. "What is coming to pass with thee, amigo mio?"

"What time is it?" I asked him.

Don Guillermo replied, "Half past one."

I turned to him. "That's a lie," I shouted. "Another one of your dirty tricks to break me down."

He nodded to Don Pedro. I caught a glimpse of two brown-frocked men standing behind him in the doorway. In a flash my mind was made up. Although I knew this was useless, I dashed for the other door leading to the small room where I had met Valerie yesterday.

"Roberto. Senor Goulet. Friend of mine. Amigo. Senor Roberto."

It seemed that everybody was calling me at the same time, and from all directions at once, as I opened the door and came face to face with two more brown-frocked attendants blocking my escape. Then all of a sudden everybody was silent, staring at me. The only thing I could do was to stare back dumbly, counting the faces, then finding a spark of hope in realising that there were only five. "Six attendants are needed for a shock treatment," I thought. "So maybe this is merely the second part of Don Guillermo's test."

"Come along, senor," he said, and took one step in my direction.

"Roberto," Don Pedro said kindly, coming towards me. "Listen, friend of mine. This is for your own good. It does not hurt at all. You will feel nothing. I promise."

I stepped back, till I could feel my shoulders against the wall. Then I saw the five of them forming a half circle slowly closing in on me. "No," I shouted. "You cannot do that to me."

"And why not?" said Don Guillermo. He spread his arms sideways in a motion to the others to stop where they were.

"Because you can't, that's all. It is against the law. You haven't asked my wife's permission. And what about my consul?"

"You are a very sick man, senor Roberto. It is our duty to treat you. We need nobody's permission. Now come on your own. Otherwise we shall have to take you by force."

"No," I shouted, now pleading against my will. "I don't want to. I'm afraid."

"But there is nothing to fear," Don Pedro said. "It does not hurt at all, Roberto."

"It is the effect I'm afraid of," I went on, desperate to the point of tears and feeling the dark rage rising up in me. "I'm afraid I will never be able to write again."

"Que va!" Don Guillermo exclaimed. "You will write even better afterwards. There will be less violence in you."

I caught the thin smile on his lips as he said this. And once again I knew it was between him and me, to

138

the bitter end. "I need my violence," I said. "I need my obsessions, all of them. You can't take that away from me. That's all I have."

Don Pedro shook his head sadly. There was an exchange of looks between Don Guillermo and the other attendants. Don Pedro stepped towards me.

"Don't," I pleaded, pushing back against the wall.

His hand dropped. The other attendants came closer, the four of them. I saw Don Guillermo stepping back towards his desk. The only thought in my mind was to leap past the attendants and grab him, then hold him till he let me free, or kill him before he could kill me.

But all of a sudden my hands and arms were being held by a thousand fingers digging into my skin and muscles, and it felt as if my bones would break if I made the least effort to move. I could not breathe. I felt burning hot all over. My feet left the ground.

Now the wall was no longer there to support my back. The sneering face of Don Guillermo seemed to drop out of sight. I saw a stretch of white ceiling rolling past. I knew I was trying to kick and scream and free my hands and arms. Not a sound came out of the attendants. There was nothing but the whitewashed ceiling rolling past overhead, then a turn, now several dark beams, and now a window with bars rising to the level of my sight.

I remember all those brown-frocked men bending over and holding me down. I remember the cool contact of jelly on my temples. I remember a sudden opening at last through the maze of arms over my chest, and Don Guillermo's face. I remember a last agonizing effort to grab him, then holding him tight, tight against a sudden attack of pain in my arms and shoulders and wrists, holding tight until I felt nothing, knew nothing but that I had him now and we would kill each other at the same time since that was what he wanted.

Suddenly there was nothing more to feel, or to know.

AN EPILOGUE

That is how it was.

If this were fiction I would now tell you how it ended. But this being a true story I can no more control the ending than tell the future. There is no certainty that I shall always resist the enchantment of alienation. I am still very much afraid to lose my mind, at times, and this strange fear is touched with a quality of hope such as I have known only on the threshold of falling in love. How long this will last, I do not know. Writing this narrative was supposed to have some therapeutic value. It has not worked out that way. Too much of me still clings to the notion that I may have never left the Manicomio.

Yet I was released, after three days, and in pretty much the same circumstances Alfredo had outlined.

Our special doctor was true to Alfredo's sketch of him. We all met on the steps of the courthouse, he cast an approving look at Valerie, steadied the carnation in his buttonhole, searched the white of my eyes a moment, then asked what I had gotten so drunk for. Work, I told him. He shook his head, bowed to Valerie and said with a twinkle in his eye. "A beautiful woman is the only valid reason for a man to end up in a manicomio." We then chatted a while about the beauties of Mallorca. I was careful not to mention Cala

D'Or. He asked if we intended to stay on the island. We said yes, as long as we could. Whereupon he said to Alfredo, "I formally declare this gentleman to be perfectly sane." It all seemed so unreal.

The High Court judge was as sympathetic as Alfredo had said he would be. What had happened in Fornalutx did not seem to interest him at all. It was my remarks about Franco and the Guardia Civil that held his attention. He asked if my insults were meant as a criticism of the political situation in Spain, and if not, why I had chosen such a figure of speech. My reply was that I did not remember what I had said. He nodded that he understood, then asked if I owned a home and if I liked living in Mallorca. I said yes twice, careful not to add anything from fear of saying the wrong thing. The judge then stood up, and, addressing Alfredo, declared I was a free man. It was hard to believe.

When we go to Palma, nowadays, I sometimes leave Valerie to her shopping and then take a taxi to the Manicomio where I give Sor Catalina some fruit and cigarettes for my old friends. Approaching the place, I usually know an instant of excitement, as on the edge of finding something I lost, then driving away always makes me feel a bit sad, as if I had left something behind. More curious still, though I usually have a good sense of direction, and after all the times I have been to the Manicomio already, I still do not know how to get there from Palma.